Dear Art

With gratitude and
appreciation to all your
support.

Much LOVE

20, Aug, 05

DISASTER AND MASS TRAUMA

GLOBAL PERSPECTIVES ON POST-DISASTER

MENTAL HEALTH MANAGEMENT

DR. ANIE SANENTZ KALAYJIAN

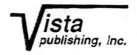

Vista publishing, Inc.

Contributing Editors: Jerena Burdge-Rezvan, Dr. Diane Dettmore, Ara Baruyr Sanentz, Shahé Navasart Sanentz, Joseph Jaeger

Cover Design by Glazer and Kalayjian, Inc.
            in collaboration with Thomas Taylor of Thomcatt Graphics

Vista Publishing, Inc.
473 Broadway
Long Branch, NJ 07750
(908) 229-6500

This publication is designed to provide information with regard to the subject matter covered. It is based on the experience and expertise of the author and is not intended to be the sole source of expertise on the subject matter. All opinions are that of the author. This book is sold with the understanding of the reader that if further information is required, the reader will seek additional sources of expert information.

Printed and bound in the United States of America

ISBN: 1-880245-32-8
Library of Congress Catalog Card Number: 95-61475

First Edition

U.S.A. Price $29.95
Canada Price $35.95

SPECIAL THANKS

TO THE FOLLOWING GUEST CONTRIBUTORS

KATHLEEN ALLDEN, MD; JOYCE BRAAK, MD;
JOEL OSLER BRENDE, MD; YAEL DANIELI, PhD; CHRIS DUNNING, PhD;
CALVIN J. FREDERICK, PhD; EDMUND L. GERGERIAN, MD;
MARY GRACE, MEd, MS; BONNIE L. GREEN, PhD;
HAIKAZ GRIGORIAN, MD;
DURAND F. JACOBS, PhD; LEVON N. JERNAZIAN, PhD;
MELINE KARAKASHIAN, PhD; BARBARA KAZANIS, CET, EdD;
DIANE KUPELIAN, PhD; JACOB LINDY, MD; RICHARD MERCER, PhD;
ELIZABETH PUCKETT, BA; JAMES R. WILL

GUEST CONTRIBUTORS
AFFILIATIONS

Kathleen Allden, MD
Dr. Allden is the Director of the Indochinese Psychiatric Clinic (IPC) located at the Deaconess Hospital in Boston, Massachusetts. She also serves as the Medical Director of the Harvard Program in Refugee Trauma (HPRT).

Joyce Braak, MD
Dr. Braak is a Psychiatrist currently practicing at Cabrini Medical Center in New York City.

Joel Osler Brende, MD
Dr. Brende is Clinical Driector of the Regional Psychiatric Division at Central State Hospital in Milledgeville, Georgia.

Yael Danieli, PhD
Dr. Danieli is currently practicing as a Clinical Psychologist in New York City.

Chris Dunning, PhD
Dr. Dunning is Professor and Chair of the Department of Governmental Affairs at the University of Wisconsin, Milwakee, Wisconsin.

Calvin J. Frederick, PhD
Dr. Frederick serves as Professor, Department of Psychiatry and Behavorial Sciences Center at U.C.L.A. School of Health, Los Angeles, California.

Edmund L. Gergerian, MD
Dr. Gergerian serves as the Chief of Psychiatry at the Staten Island Developmental Disabilities Center in Staten Island, New York.

Mary Grace, Med, MS
Ms. Grace is Senior Research Associate at the University of Cincinnati, College of Medicine, Cincinnati, Ohio.

Bonnie L. Green, PhD
Dr. Green is currently serving as Professor of Psychiatry in the Department of Psychiatry at Georgetown University Hospital in Washington, DC.

Haikaz Grigorian, MD
Dr. Grigorian is an Associate Professor of Clinical Psychiatry at the University of Medicine and Dentistry of New Jersey in Newark, New Jersey.

Durand F. Jacobs, PhD
Dr. Jacobs serves as Clinical Professor of Psychiatry at the Loma Linda University Medical School in Redlands, California.

Levon N. Jernazian, PhD
Dr. Jernazian is an Instructor of Psychology at the Gelndale Community College in Gelndale, California.

Meline Karakashian, PhD
Dr. Karakashian is currently the Clinical Psychologist for the Old Bridge Township School system in New Jersey.

Barbara Kazanis, CET, EdD
Dr. Kazanis is the Direcotr of the Life Center, Center for the Arts and Human Development, University of South Florida, Tampa, Florida.

Diane Kupelian, PhD
Dr. Kupelian is a practicing Clinical Psychologist in Bethesda, Maryland.

Jacob Lindy, MD
Dr. Lindy is the Director of the Cincinnati Center for Psychoanlysis in Cincinnati, Ohio.

Richard G. Mercer, PhD
Dr. Mercer is a Clinical Psychologist and Director of the Department of Veterans Affairs Medical Center, Newark, New Jersey.

Elizabeth Puckett, BA
Ms. Puckett is the Coordinator of Cooperative for Assistance and Relief Everywhere (CARE) located in Atlanta, Georgia.

James L. Will
Mr. Will is the Director of the Federal Emergency Management Agency (FEMA) in Washington, DC.

MEET THE AUTHOR

Dr. Anie Sanentz Kalayjian is an educator, international trauma expert, logotherapeutic psychotherapist, registered professional nurse, researcher, and consultant. She has over ten years of experience in disaster management and mass trauma intervention. She has over fifteen years of clinical experience and university teaching.

Dr. Sanentz Kalayjian holds Master's and Doctoral degrees from Teachers College, Columbia University and has completed several post-graduate courses at the William Alanson White Institute. She is certified by the American Nurses Credentialing Center in Psychiatric and Mental Health Nursing Practice, and holds an advanced Certificate from the American Red Cross in disaster management, and an advanced Certificate in Eye Movement Desensitization and Reprocessing (EMDR). She is a Dutch Diplomate in Logotherapy and is a candidate for the American Diplomate in Logotherapy.

In the area of man-made disasters, she has worked extensively with veterans of the Gulf and Vietnam Wars, Holocaust survivors, and Armenian survivors of the Ottoman Turkish Genocide. In the area of natural disasters, she has worked extensively with the survivors of the 1988 earthquake in Armenia, of the 1994 earthquake of southern California, of hurricane Andrew in southern Florida, and of the 1995 earthquake in Kobe, Japan. Dr. Sanentz Kalayjian has assisted mental health professionals in Kuwait and the former Yugoslavia as a consultant.

For the past three years, Dr. Sanentz Kalayjian has been actively involved in the United Nations, pursuing the human rights of children, survivors of disasters, women and refugees. She is the World Federation for Mental Health representative for the United Nations, Secretary/Treasurer of the NGO Committee for Human Rights, a member of the UNICF working group on Exploited Children, a member of the NGO Committee on the Status of Women, and a member of the Fourth World Conference on Women's working group on Women and Mental Health. She is also the official delegate of the World Federation for Mental Health to the Fourth World Conference on Women held in Beijing, China.

Dr. Sanentz Kalayjian is founder and President of the Armenian American Society for Studies on Stress and Genocide, vice-president of the International Society for Traumatic Stress Studies, New York Chapter, and the Chairperson of the Education Committee of the New York Counties Registered Nurses Association.

Dr. Sanentz Kalayjian is co-founder of the Mental Health Outreach Program to the Republic of Armenia, providing care, managing the program, as well as conducting research. The outreach program has since been implemented in Kuwait and the former Yugoslavia.

Dr. Sanentz Kalayjian is a recipient of numerous scholarships and awards, among them: the Clark Foundation Scholarship Award, the Endowed Nursing Scholarship, the Professor Traineeship from Columbia University, the Armenian Students' Association Scholarship, the Armenian Relief Society Scholarship, the Honorary Dutch Diplomate in Logotherapy, 1993 Research and Scholarship Award from Teachers College, and honors from the American Psychological Association and the New York Counties Registered Nurses Association. She has also been the recipient of the Jane Delano Distinguished Service Award, American Psychological Association, and the ABSA Outstanding Achievement Award. Dr. Sanentz Kalayjian was inducted as an honorary member of Kappa Delta Pi, and Sigma Theta Tau. She is listed in *Who's Who Among Students in American Colleges and Universities*, *Who's Who of American Women*, the *Armenian Women at Work*, *Who's Who Among Armenians*, *Distinguished Leader*, and the *World Who's Who of Women*.

Dr. Sanentz Kalayjian is an active member of many professional organizations, among them: Fellow of the American Orthopsychiatric Association, the Association of the Training Institute for Mental Health Practitioners, Council on Continuing Education, and the Council on Psychiatric and Mental Health Nursing. In addition, she is an active member of the Institute of Logotherapy, Society for Educational Research in Psychiatric and Mental Health Nursing, the Association of University Professors, American Nurses' Association, and the International Society for Traumatic Stress Studies.

Dr. Sanentz Kalayjian has presented her research papers, conducted workshops, and chaired panel discussions nationwide. Internationally, her research papers have been presented in the Republic of Armenia, Canada, Finland, France, Italy, Japan, Korea, Mexico, Moscow, the Middle East, the Netherlands, Spain, and Taiwan. She maintains ongoing collaborative research projects with the Republic of Armenia, the Netherlands, Moscow, and Japan.

She has published nationally and internationally in various scholarly and professional journals and has several chapters in a variety of books to her credit. Dr. Sanentz Kalayjian has been interviewed on television and the radio in the United States and abroad.

ACKNOWLEDGMENTS

This manual is dedicated to all those survivors with whom I have worked in both natural and man-made disasters, including but not limited to: my father and other Armenian survivors of the Ottoman Turkish Genocide, the survivors of the earthquakes in Southern California, San Francisco, and the Republic of Armenia, the survivors of the Hurricane Andrew in Southern Florida; and the survivors of the Gulf War in Kuwait. Their experiences help advance the science and art of caring and help refine the science of disaster management.

I thank all the expert contributors to this manual, who have been my mentors, role models, and colleagues. Special thanks to all those who worked collaboratively to collect data and provided access to their institutions, especially to Mrs. Gail Gordon, Director of Nursing, and her dedicated staff at South Miami Hospital - Homestead, who worked to facilitate the research process.

Finally, I thank my husband Shahe N. Sanentz, my brother-in-law Ara B. Sanentz and my friends, Dr. Harold Takooshian and Robert Lee Jones for all their editorial support and constructive criticism.

FORWARD

BY

Jacob D. Lindy, MD

Each year the human and material consequences of natural disaster grow more severe. Advances in technology, while improving our warning systems and efficiency of relief efforts, shield us from realizing that, worldwide, the tragic human problems from natural disaster are expanding, not receding.

Prominent in the effects of these natural disasters are the acute and long term emotional reactions which characterize individuals and communities. In this book, Anie Kalayjian and her colleagues describe the nature of such reactions as they pertain to three recent disasters, the Armenian earthquake, the South Florida hurricane and the Los Angeles earthquake. The book also describes in a state-of-th- art manner the planning and delivery of mental health services, as well as the research and new understandings gained from studying the mental health response to these tragedies.

It is important to realize that for much of this century, mental health effects of natural disaster were not generally acknowledged. Roy Popkin, director of the Red Cross observed in his introduction to Murphy and Laube's *Perspectives on Disaster Recovery*, that in the past, professionals who were central to the disaster recovery effort ignored the psychological dimension "simply because the experts told us so." As a result, clinical observations and interventions were not systematic and no general body of mental health related clinical knowledge had been accumulating or could be integrated with the tasks of other disaster workers.

In the past twenty years, the area of disaster and psychological trauma has taken wings. Mardi Hoorowitz's seminal work on the intrusive and denial phases of post traumatic reactions set the stage for pooling knowledge from natural disaster trauma with industrial trauma and war trauma. With the introduction of post traumatic stress disorder as a designated entity in the official psychiatric nomenclature in 1980, this entity has received systematic attention from a variety of clinical and theoretical fields. Whereas no standardized instruments existed twenty years ago, today the worker in the field is confronted with a variety of measurements, and needs to select carefully the ones that are most suitable.

The purview of earlier collected works is limited to the USA and the Caribbeans. In this volume the dialogue between West and East which was part of perestroika and the radical changes in Eastern Europe and Russia are implicit in the pages of the book. American trauma therapists working beside Armenian and Russian colleagues was laying the groundwork for more widespread interactions yet to come.

Further, through informal electronic networks, communication moves quickly from workers at one disaster site to the next. Indeed, today's disasters occur in the context of a global community.

In contrast to the past, today's mental health professionals and specially trained non-professionals see it as their duty to provide care; social supports are worked with in a planful manner; a wide variety of interventions are available, thoughtful outreach is planned and careful research is conducted.

While paying careful attention to earlier perspectives, the current book expands them in important ways such as the need to prepare and care for the disaster's impact on the helpers themselves.

Thus, each of the newer elements in the mental health dimension to post disaster care which have arisen in the last quarter century is part of Dr. Kalayjian's monograph.

Anie Kalayjian, in the tradition of earlier monographs by Parad Resnik and Parad, Souder, Lystad, and Laube and Murphy, emphasizes a model which integrates practical aspects of post disaster care; she and her selected authors are never far from a hands-on perspective.

Dr. Kalayjian organizes this monograph around a series of practical steps, ones which she found to be useful in delivering care to the survivors of the Armenian earthquake and has named the Mental Health Outreach Program. The six steps inform the intervention team about the historical and sociological forces at work pre-disaster, the impact of the catastrophe itself, and analysis of consequences , an assessment of how to implement the most salient interventions, evaluate them, and remodify the plan on the basis of this evaluation.

She helps the reader digest an array of topics by focusing in a practical way by keeping illustrations from three specific disasters close to the reader's attention.

Practical management or mismanagement of disaster often involves the interworkings of various helping agencies. Distinctions in mission, priorities and jurisdiction have traditionally left gaps and redundancies in care. By bringing leaders of these organizations into the authorship of this book she underlines the importance of the interrelatedness of these perspectives.

While featuring the most up-to-date psychological and biophysiological interventions, there is a unifying organization to the therapeutic activity which she chooses to review. Each intervention mode attends to one of the following crucial needs of survivors: expressing emotion, containing overstimulation, seeking support, and searching for meaning.

A context of symptom distress, adaptation and meaning provides the underlying texture for the book. Integrating older models (e.g. crisis intervention) with newer modalities and perspectives (such as PTSD research, biophysiological and existential) she keeps the focus on the meaning of the experience to individual people and their lives.

Disaster and Mass Trauma, Global Perspectives On Post-Disaster Mental Health Management, while taking a broad view, retains the personal subjective view of survivors who are overwhelmed, unprepared, grieved, in despair and angry, and of survivors who find their exposure to tragedy, hope, redefinition of identity and new commitment to life. This book is the next necessary building block in our library of knowledge regarding mental health and disaster.

EARTHQUAKE IN ARMENIA

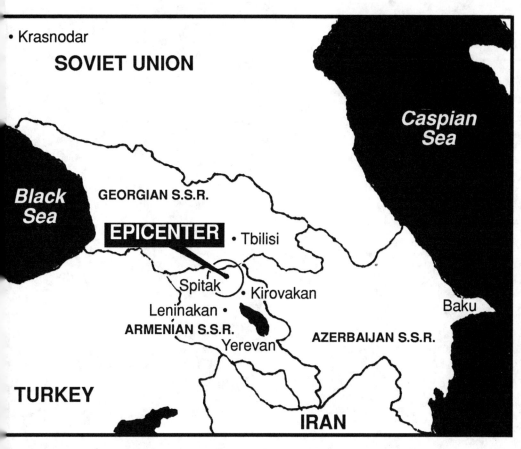

- Krasnodar
  SOVIET UNION
  Caspian Sea
  Black Sea
  GEORGIAN S.S.R.
  EPICENTER • Tbilisi
  Spitak
  • Kirovakan
  Leninakan •
  ARMENIAN S.S.R.
  Baku
  Yerevan
  AZERBAIJAN S.S.R.
  TURKEY
  IRAN

December 7, 1988

Path Of Hurricane Andrew

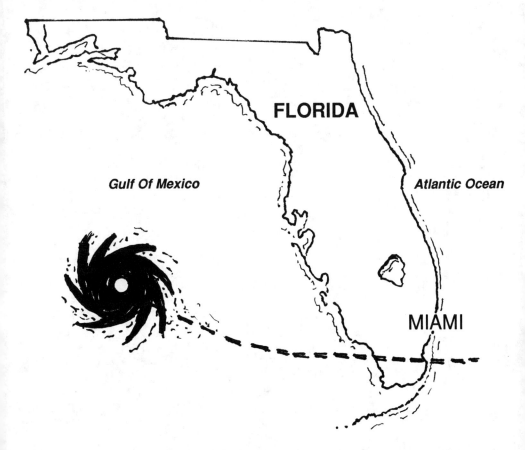

SOUTH FLORIDA, AUGUST 24, 1992

Los Angeles Earthquake
JANUARY 17, 1994

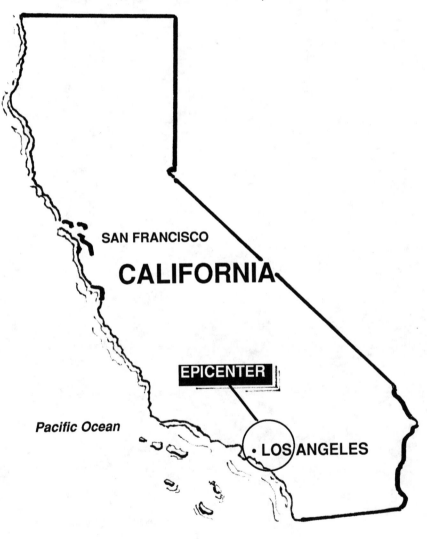

SAN FRANCISCO

CALIFORNIA

EPICENTER

Pacific Ocean

· LOS ANGELES

TABLE OF CONTENTS

TABLE OF CONTENTS

TABLE OF CONTENTS

TABLE OF CONTENTS

Appendices

CHAPTER I

INTRODUCTION AND OVERVIEW

CHAPTER I

The birth of all things is weak and tender,
and therefore,
we should have our eyes intent on beginnings.

Montague, 1580-1588

INTRODUCTION
and
OVERVIEW

Natural disasters, scientists agree, are unavoidable.   Earthquakes, hurricanes, tidal waves, floods and fires can occur anywhere. During the last decade, devastating earthquakes struck in Coalinga, San Francisco, the San Fernando Valley in California, Idaho, Guinea in West Africa, Liege in Belgium, Turkey, Japan, the Philippines, Hawaii, Armenia, Georgia, Mexico, Indonesia and India. Other natural disasters such as floods in Mississippi, brush fires in California, typhoons in Japan, hurricanes in South Carolina and southern Florida and tsunamis (tidal waves) in Japan, also occurred within the last decade (see Table 1). No region of the world can be considered safe or exempt from these disasters. Furthermore, the statistically-calculated trends over the last two decades indicate that both the number and the magnitude of the effects of natural disasters will continue to increase at a rapid rate in the near future (see Figures 1, 2, 3, 4). The top four natural disasters causing the most damage around the world, from 1963-1992, in the order of highest frequency, are floods, tropical storms, droughts and earthquakes. The top four disasters causing the most casualties are floods, tropical storms, epidemics and earthquakes (see Figure 5). Southern Asia and Eastern Asia are the highest hit regions (see Figure 6).

The World Health Organization (WHO) estimates that between the years 1964 and 1983, natural disasters throughout the world killed nearly 2,500,000 people and left an additional 750,000,000 injured, homeless, or otherwise affected (PAHO, 1993). The United Nations General Assembly adopted a resolution declaring the 1990's the International Decade of Natural Disaster Reduction and the U.S. Senate and House of Representatives endorsed the Decade concept in resolutions passed the following year (see Table 2). The U.S. National Committee for the International Decade for Natural Disaster Reduction (IDNDR) was formed

MAJOR DISASTERS AROUND THE WORLD, 1963-1992

Significant Disasters Based On: Damage, Persons Affected, Number Of Deaths

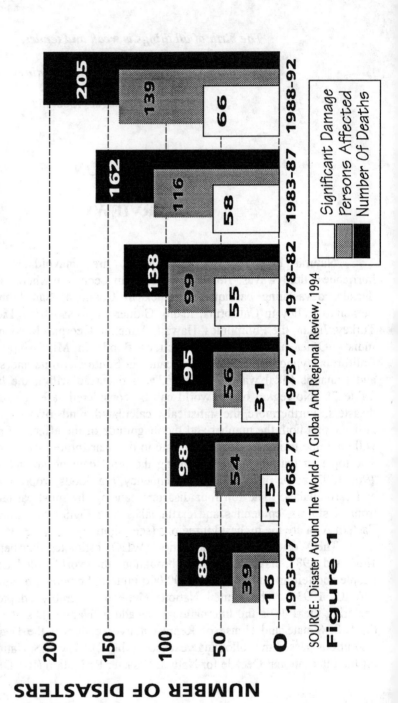

SOURCE: Disaster Around The World- A Global And Regional Review, 1994

Figure 1

MAJOR DISASTERS AROUND THE WORLD, 1963-1992

TRENDS: Number Of Significant Disasters By Category

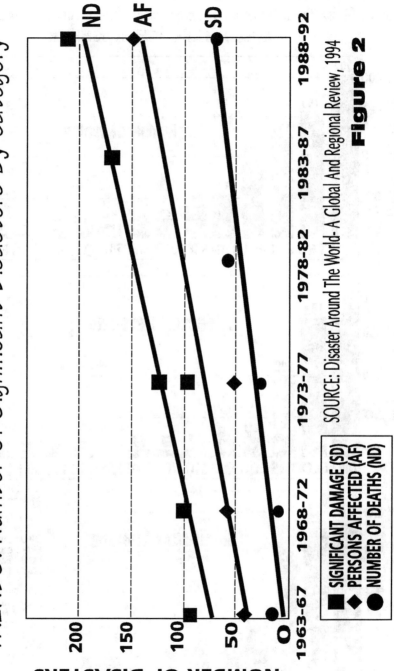

SOURCE: Disaster Around The World- A Global And Regional Review, 1994

Figure 2

MAJOR DISASTERS AROUND THE WORLD

Number Of Significant Disasters By Type: Damage, Persons Affected, Number Of Deaths

SOURCE: Disaster Around The World, - A Global And Regional Review, 1994

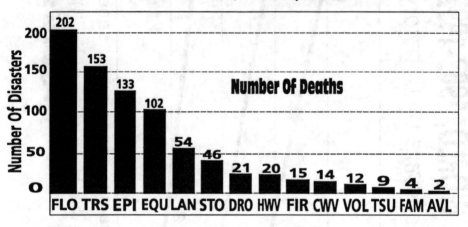

Number Of Deaths

FLO	TRS	EPI	EQU	LAN	STO	DRO	HWV	FIR	CWV	VOL	TSU	FAM	AVL
202	153	133	102	54	46	21	20	15	14	12	9	4	2

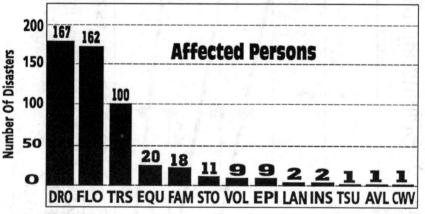

Affected Persons

DRO	FLO	TRS	EQU	FAM	STO	VOL	EPI	LAN	INS	TSU	AVL	CWV
167	162	100	20	18	11	9	9	2	2	1	1	1

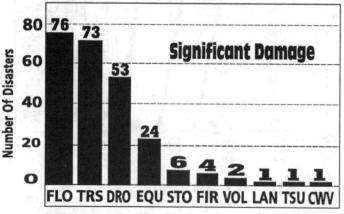

Significant Damage

FLO	TRS	DRO	EQU	STO	FIR	VOL	LAN	TSU	CWV
76	73	53	24	6	4	2	1	1	1

KEY
AVL• Avalanches
CWV• Cold Waves
DRO• Drought
EPI• Epidemics
EQU• Earthquakes
FAM• Food Shortages
        Famine
FIR• Fires
FLO• Floods
HWV• Heat Waves
INS• Insect Infest
LAN• Landslides
STO• Storms, Other
TRS• Tropical Storms
TSU• Tsunamis
VOL• Volcanos

Figure 3

4

MAJOR DISASTERS AROUND THE WORLD, 1963-1992

% Of Significant Disasters By Type: Damage, Persons Affected, Number Of Deaths

SOURCE: Diaster Around The World - A Global And Regional Review, 1994

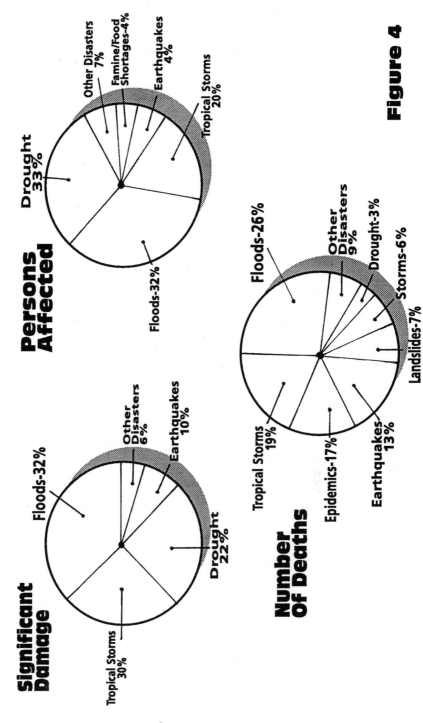

Persons Affected

Drought 33%

Other Disasters 7%

Famine/Food Shortages-4%

Earthquakes 4%

Tropical Storms 20%

Floods-32%

Significant Damage

Floods-32%

Other Disasters 6%

Earthquakes 10%

Drought 22%

Tropical Storms 30%

Number Of Deaths

Floods-26%

Other Disasters 9%

Drought-3%

Storms-6%

Landslides-7%

Tropical Storms 19%

Epidemics-17%

Earthquakes 13%

Figure 4

5

MAJOR DISASTERS AROUND THE WORLD, 1963-1992
Trends: Most Significant Disaster Types By Category

SOURCE: Disaster Around The World, - A Global And Regional Review, 1994

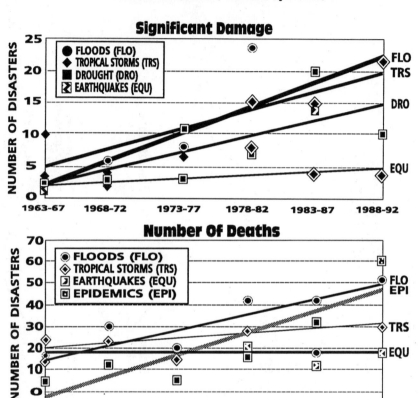

Significant Damage

NUMBER OF DISASTERS

- ● FLOODS (FLO)
- ◆ TROPICAL STORMS (TRS)
- ■ DROUGHT (DRO)
- ▨ EARTHQUAKES (EQU)

FLO
TRS
DRO
EQU

1963-67 1968-72 1973-77 1978-82 1983-87 1988-92

Number Of Deaths

NUMBER OF DISASTERS

- ● FLOODS (FLO)
- ◈ TROPICAL STORMS (TRS)
- ▨ EARTHQUAKES (EQU)
- ▣ EPIDEMICS (EPI)

FLO
EPI
TRS
EQU

1963-67 1968-72 1973-77 1978-82 1983-87 1988-92

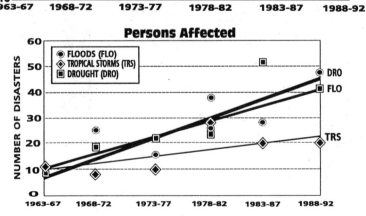

Persons Affected

NUMBER OF DISASTERS

- ● FLOODS (FLO)
- ◈ TROPICAL STORMS (TRS)
- ■ DROUGHT (DRO)

DRO
FLO
TRS

1963-67 1968-72 1973-77 1978-82 1983-87 1988-92

MAJOR DISASTERS BY REGION, 1963-1992

Regional Comparison - Disasters By Category - Entire Period

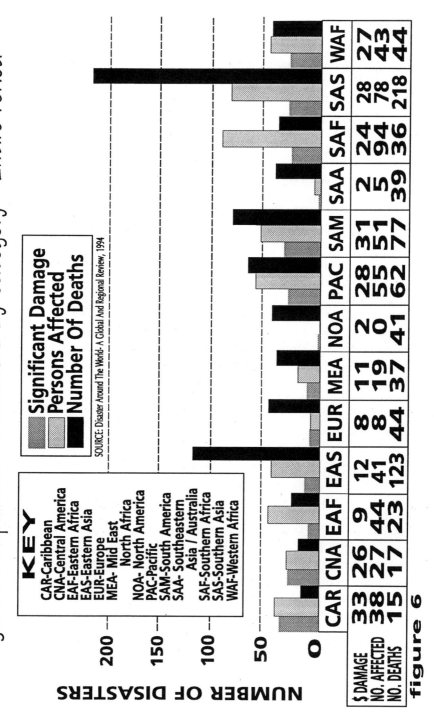

KEY

CAR-Caribbean
CNA-Central America
EAF-Eastern Africa
EAS-Eastern Asia
EUR-Europe
MEA- Mid East
North Africa
NOA- North America
PAC-Pacific
SAM-South America
SAA- Southeastern
Asia / Australia
SAF-Southern Africa
SAS-Southern Asia
WAF-Western Africa

Significant Damage
Persons Affected
Number Of Deaths

SOURCE: Disaster Around The World- A Global And Regional Review, 1994

	CAR	CNA	EAF	EAS	EUR	MEA	NOA	PAC	SAM	SAA	SAF	SAS	WAF
$ DAMAGE	33	26	9	12	8	11	2	28	31	2	24	28	27
NO. AFFECTED	38	27	44	41	8	19	0	55	51	5	94	78	43
NO. DEATHS	15	17	23	123	44	37	41	62	77	39	36	218	44

NUMBER OF DISASTERS

figure 6

7

to provide encouragement to government agencies as well as private groups and individuals to be involved in relevant disaster reduction activities. Members of the National Committee are as follows:

1. Walter Lynn (Chair), Cornell University, Ithaca, New York
2. Lawrence Grossman, Horizons TV, New York, New York
3. George Housner, California Institute of Technology, Pasadena, California
4. Shirley Mattingly, Los Angeles, California
5. Gordon Eaton, U.S. Geological Survey, Washington, DC
6. E.L. (Henry) Quarantelli, University of Delaware, Newark, Delaware
7. Kathryn Sullivan, National Oceanic and Atmospheric Administration, Washington, DC
8. James Lee Witt, Federal Emergency Management Agency, Washington, DC

The Decade of Natural Disaster Reduction has inspired many professionals to educate the community in disaster management. In 1994, the United Nations World Conference on Natural Disaster Reduction in Yokohama, Japan attempted to review and recognize the mid-decade efforts and accomplishments of each participating nation. The World Conference attempted also to increase commitment to accomplishing the goals set forth for the Decade.

Following the 1994 World Conference, the National Committee presented a report encompassing the following views and perspectives about how the United States has addressed the IDNDR targets:

1. Risk Assessment:

Risk assessment involves assessing the vulnerability of a region. Many of the hazard-prone areas in the United States are generally known, for example, the coastlines, which are vulnerable to hurricanes, flooding and erosion. Progress has also been made in the identified earthquake belts, but information is still insufficient to accurately determine the risk in many areas. Loss of life due to natural disasters in the United States has decreased steadily and this loss is much lower than in other countries where there may be a natural disaster event of similar magnitude. For example, whereas the 1988 earthquake in Armenia, which measured 6.9 on the Richter scale, caused approximately 75,000 estimated casualties, the 1994 earthquake in Northridge, California, which also measured 6.9 on the Richter scale, resulted in 61 deaths. And, though the 1994 earthquake in Colombia, which measured 8.2 on the Richter scale, caused 1,000 deaths, the 1989 earthquake in Loma Prieta, California, caused approximately 63 deaths. The

United States has reduced threats to human lives and personal injury through more effective warning systems, disaster education and preparedness.

2. Mitigation:

Although mitigation has been a requirement of Federal emergency management policy for about 30 years in the United States, many highly vulnerable states remain without building codes to ensure wind resistance, as in South Carolina, which experienced major damage from Hurricane Hugo in 1989. Some States do have the building codes but do not enforce them, e.g., Dade County, Florida, evidenced by the vast destruction observed after Hurricane Andrew in 1992.

During the remainder of the Decade, Federal agencies plan to elevate mitigation as a priority in their disaster reduction programs. The U.S. Federal Emergency Management Agency (FEMA), in particular, is developing a National Mitigation Strategy as a priority for the next century. It is a challenge to involve all levels of the administration, as well as the private sector, in these mitigation plans.

3. Warning Systems:

The United Statesspends billions of dollars on maintenance and improvement of systems to detect, monitor, and disseminate information regarding natural disasters. Dissemination of essential information to developing countries is essential. Over the last 40 years, the reduction in the number of lives lost each year due to natural disasters is partly due to advancement in detection, warning systems, and dissemination of this information. The overwhelming number of casualties in Armenia was largely caused by poor information processing, lack of organization, and an absence of warning and evacuation procedures.

According to the U.S. National Committee Report (1994), although loss of life due to natural disasters in the United States has decreased, economic losses are on the rise. These economic losses are comprised of losses to property, infrastructure damage and loss of revenues and resources. The 1989 earthquake in Loma Prieta, California caused 63 deaths and $8 billion in damages; in contrast, the 1994 earthquake in Northridge, California caused fewer deaths (57), but more than double in estimated damages ($20 billion). Also according to the Report, more than half of the U.S. population lives in coastal zones or along fault lines, and surprisingly, most of the population growth is taking place there. This is an interesting phenomenon to research, as most of the population is oblivious to the hazards to which they are exposed. This author raises the question as to the true level of awareness of the population as opposed to the potential existence of

How many EARTHQUAKES are located each year?

Table 1
Number of earthquakes located worldwide
from 1984 to 1993 by the USGS/NEIC

Magnitude	1984	1985	1986	1987	1988	1989	1990	1991	1992	1993
8.0 to 9.9	0	1	1	0	0	1	0	0	0	1
7.0 to 7.9	8	13	5	11	8	6	12	11	23	15
6.0 to 6.9	91	110	89	112	93	79	115	105	104	141
5.0 to 5.9	1579	1674	1665	1437	1485	1444	1635	1469	1541	1449
4.0 to 4.9	3683	4281	4476	4146	4018	4090	4493	4372	5196	5034
3.0 to 3.9	1579	1764	1942	1806	1932	2452	2457	2952	4643	4263
2.0 to 2.9	442	935	1169	1037	1479	1906	2364	2927	3068	5390
1.0 to 1.9	37	97	153	102	118	418	474	801	887	1177
0.1 to 0.9	0	0	0	0	3	0	0	1	2	9
unknown	3074	4240	3218	2639	3575	4189	5062	3878	4084	3997
Total	**10493**	**13115**	**12718**	**11290**	**12711**	**14585**	**16612**	**16516**	**19548**	**21476**

Table 2
Frequency of occurrence of earthquakes
based on observations since 1900

Descriptor	Magnitude	Average Annually
Great	8 and higher	1
Major	7-7.9	18
Strong	6-6.9	120
Moderate	5-5.9	800
Light	4-4.9	6,200 (estimated)
Minor	3-3.9	49,000 (estimated)
Very Minor	less than 3	Mag. 2-3: about 1,000/day Mag. 1-2: about 8,000/day

Prepared by The U.S. Geological Survey's National Earthquake Information Center

denial, a death wish (Thanatos) or ignorance of those living in these potential disaster zones.

The number of natural disasters around the world continues to grow. According to the U.S. Geological Survey's National Earthquake Information Center, there were 10,493 earthquakes in 1984. This number had more then doubled in 1993 with 21, 476 (see table 1). Therefore, frequency of occurrence of earthquakes daily of less than 3 magnitude are about 9,000 (see table 2). In quite a few developing countries, total annual losses from natural disasters exceeded the amount of international assistance provided to them. A recent study, reported at the World Conference in Japan 1994, has shown that in the last two decades the number of persons affected by these disasters was increasing at the rate of 6% per year, which corresponds to three times the annual population growth.

HURRICANE ANDREW

South Florida • August 24, 1992

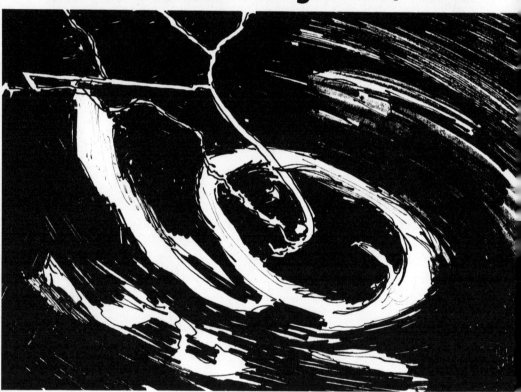

DEFINITIONS

We read the world wrong and say it deceives us.

Tagore, from Stray Birds, LXXV

Disaster:

Although the lay public loosely defines the term disaster as a dangerous, sudden, and uncontrollable situation, researchers and practitioners are less in consensus as to a disaster's definition, characteristics and effects on mental health (Quarantelli, 1985; Tierney, 1986). Tierney (1989) defined the term as collective stress in a particular geographic area interfering with the ongoing social life of the community, with a sudden onset, some degree of loss and subject to human management. Other experts (Quarantelli, 1970; Stallings, 1973; Warheit, 1976) distinguish between natural disasters in which there is a community consensus and civil disturbances in which there is dissensus. Quarantelli (1985) distinguishes a disaster from a conflict (e.g., riots, hostages, incidents), and a community disaster from a group disaster (e.g., train derailment, sinking ship or aircraft crash).

According to the Pan American Health Organization (PAHO) Regional Office of the World Health Organization (WHO) (1993), disasters are defined as events occurring suddenly, in most cases, and which cause severe disturbances in the community. Those disturbances could be in the form of loss of life, health, or resources; and in the form of disruption: of life, of environmental quality, as well as socio-economic disruptions requiring immediate and comprehensive assistance and a variety of interventions. From 1988-1995 damages due to natural disasters have been valued at $100 billion dollars (see Table 4). Disasters are classified as: natural, man-made, and hybrid (see Table 3).

This author differentiates personal disasters from collective ones. In a personal disaster, one unit of the community is affected by the incident, such as an automobile accident affecting one family. This manual will address collective natural disasters, where more than one unit of the community is affected or a situation which challenges the existing resources of the community that makes outside interventions absolutely essential for its future viability. As the U.N. Secretary General Boutros Boutros-Ghali stated in his address to the IDNDR Special High-Level Council in January, 1993, *"There is no hard and fast division - in terms of their effects on civilian population - between conflicts and wars, and natural disasters. Droughts, floods, earthquakes and cyclones are just as destructive for communities and settlements as wars and civil confrontation."*

Disaster Classification and Predominant Agent

Table 3

Disaster Type	Natural	Man-Made	Hybrid
Avalanche/Rockfall	Yes	No	Yes
Landslide/Mudslide	Yes	Yes	Yes
Transport			
•Air	No	Yes	Yes
•Road	No	Yes	Yes
•Marine	No	Yes	Yes
•Rail	No	Yes	Yes
Climatic	Yes	No	?
Drought	Yes	Yes	Yes
Famine	Yes	Yes	Yes
Epidemic	Yes	No	Yes
Plague	Yes	Yes	Yes
Earthquake	Yes	No	No
Fire	Yes	Yes	Yes
Explosion	No	Yes	Yes
Flooding	Yes	No	Yes
Mining	No	Yes	Yes
Volcanic Activity	Yes	No	Yes
Miscellaneous	No	Yes	Yes

Source: Strategic Aspects of Geological and Seismic Disaster Management and Disaster Scenario Planning Seminar in Moscow, Alma - Ata, and Frunze, October 1990 and 1991
United Nations, Department of Humanitarian Affairs Publication, 1993
Prepared by Eric E. Alley, UNDRO Consultant

RECENT NATURAL HAZARDS

Table 4

TYPE/LOCATION				AFFECTED POPULATION/LOSSES
Hurricanes	1988	Sept.	Hurricane Gilibert, Haiti/Jamaica	$1.5 million damage
	1989		Hugo-South Carolina and Virgin Islands	49 deaths; $9 billion damage
	1992	Aug.	Andrew-Florida and Louisiana	15 deaths; $30 billion damage
	1992		Iniki-Hawaii	6 deaths; $2 billion damage
Wildfires	1990		Santa Barbara, California	0 deaths; $235 million damage
	1991		Oakland/Berkeley Hills, California	25 deaths; $1.5 billion damage
	1993		Southern California	3 deaths; $1 billion damage
Earthquake	1988	Dec.	Armenia, USSR	$500,000 damage
	1989	Oct.	Loma Prieta, California	67 deaths; $10 billion damage
	1990	June	Iran	$250,000 damage
	1990	July	Philippines	$1.5 million damage
	1994		Northridge, California	57 (estimated) deaths; $20 billion (estimated) damage
	1995	Jan.	Kobe, Japan	
Floods	1988	Aug.	Sudan	$1 million damage
	1988	Sept.	Bangladesh	$75 million damage
	1989	July	China	$100 million damage
	1989	July	Brazil	$5 million damage
	1993		Midwest (Mississippi Valley)	50 deaths; $15-20 billion damage
Volcanoes	1989		Redoubt, Alaska	1 death; less than $100 million damage
	1992		Spurr, Alaska	0 deaths; $100 million damage
Landslides	Annual Average			25 deaths; $1.5-2.5 billion damage
Tornadoes	Annual Average			100 death; $1 billion damage
Drought	Annual Average			$6-8 billion damage
Winter Storm	1994	March	USA East Coast	130 (estimated) deaths
Heat	1995	July	USA East Coast	256 deaths

NATIONAL SOCIO-ECONOMIC CONDITIONS

Population: 258,233 million (US Census, July 1993)
Gross-National Product (GNP): $5,694.9 Billion (1990 US Census)
Per-Capita Income: $14,420 (1990 US Census)

Coping difficulty:

The phase of coping difficulty includes those types of behavior which survivors perceive as a situation in which they feel helpless, uncomfortable and unable to initiate steps to resolve their difficulties.

Coping mechanism:

This phase includes patterns of responses or reactions by which the individual deals or responds to a stressor, a disaster or any hazardous event and/or crisis.

Crisis:

The word crisis has its root in the Greek word Krinein, which means to decide, separate, and judge (Random House, 1993). Crisis is indeed a special state during an ongoing process of disequilibrium whereby one has to make decisions and frequently adopt new coping mechanisms to deal with the increasing intensity of the difficulties that one encounters. A period of crisis can vary, generally lasting from one to six weeks.

Cyclone:

Cyclones are storms distinguished by low atmospheric pressure at its center. It comprises revolving winds clockwise or anti-clockwise in the southern and northern hemispheres, respectively. Cyclones are classified on the basis of the average speed of the wind near the core of the system as follows (PAHO, 1992):

Wind Speed	Classification
Up to 61KM/hr (39 mph)	Tropical Depression
61 KM/hr. (40 mph) - 115 KN/hr (73 mph)	Tropical Storm
Greater than 115 KM/hr (73 mph)	Hurricane

Earthquake:

Earthquake is a sudden motion of the ground produced by the displacement of rock masses (PAHO, 1992). It consists of a sudden release of energy due to years of accumulated stresses in parts of the earth's crust. The stresses in the crust are mainly found in the forces pulling at its component parts (the tectonic plates), which are countered by opposing forces in adjacent plates. Not much is known about these forces, but it is speculated that they may be due to the high temperatures inside the earth, as well as the force of gravity (PAHO, 1993).

The forces generated in the tectonic plates in turn produce cracks in the plates themselves, which are known as geological faults. Earthquakes caused by active geological faults are generally shallow or of intermediate depth and are therefore very dangerous (PAHO, 1993).

Additional stressors also contribute to the impact of the earthquake:

- **Mass land movement:** Landslides or collapses may happen several hours or days after the quake.

- **Ground settlement:** A phenomenon whereby loose soil itself, or lower state of soil loosened due to liquefaction or other geological causes sudden shifts.

- **Tsunami:** Also known as tidal waves. Tsunamis are gigantic ocean waves engendered by seismic events at the bottom of the ocean. A tsunami can travel thousands of miles from the epicenter of the quake, causing floods in coastal regions.

- **Liquefaction:** "A phenomenon that results in the sudden sinking of the soil because of the increase in the pressure of the water contained in the soil." (PAHO, 1993. p. 7).

- **The amplification of seismic waves by the soils:** Earthquakes occurring far from a city are practically insignificant, but they are amplified destructively when the seismic waves encounter soft soils, usually laustrine.

- **Other indirect hazards:** The force of a quake can cause cracks in dams, which, for example may contaminate an industrial plant due to leaks of gases or other dangerous substances, fires, and explosions.

Flood:

Flooding occurs either when the rate of runoff exceeds the ability of drainage facilities to cope with an intense event of a short duration or when runoff simply results from the inability of saturated substrate from absorbing furthers events of low intensity yet long duration.

Rain Fall:

Rain fall is an event of either high intensity and short duration or low intensity and long duration. It may be fed by hurricanes, tropical waves, tropical depressions, and the like.

Earthquake magnitude:

One measure of the strength of an earthquake is its magnitude as calculated from records of the event by a calibrated seismograph. Earthquake magnitude was first defined by Charles Richter in 1935 and thus named after him (PAHO, 1992).

Earthquake intensity:

Intensity is widely measured by the Modified Mercalli Intensity Scale of 12 degrees, symbolized by MM. This is a measure of the effect of the earthquake on the people, structures and the earth's surface (PAHO, 1992).

Earthquake hazards:
Two categories were identified by PAHO (1992), which are described below:

1. **Direct Hazards:**
   - Ground shaking
   - Differential ground
   - Soil liquefaction
   - Immediate landslides or mud slides, ground lurching and avalanches
   - Permanent ground displacement along faults

- Floods from tsunamis or seiches

2. <u>Indirect Hazards</u>:
   - Dam failures
   - Pollution from damage to industrial plants
   - Delayed landslides

Epicenter:

The point on the earth's surface directly above the focus where the earthquake's motion starts.

Federal:

In the United States, pertaining to the central government of the country. More generally, pertaining to a form of government in which power is divided between a set of political units and a central political entity.

Hazard:

Hazard is an unavoidable danger with the potential for risk, difficulty, trauma and a multitude of losses. The potential impact of a hazard is measured by its magnitude and intensity (PAHO, 1992). One can measure the potential hazard in a country by analyzing the area's history of natural disasters and the size, in terms of the intensities given by the Modified Mercalli Intensity Scale (PAHO, 1992).

Hurricane:

Hurricanes are violent, tropical, cyclonic storms having wind speeds of or in excess of 63 knots (72 mph, 32 m/sec) (Random House, 1993). According to PAHO (1992), a hurricane derives energy from the heat of condensation of water vapor over warm tropical seas. For a hurricane to develop there needs to be a sea temperature of at least 26° C maintained for several days, and a large expanse of sea surface, generally about 400 km, (250 miles) in diameter. Hurricanes have a unique eye - - a convenient form of reference that may be tracked by radar, aircraft, or satellite - - which has very little wind, and as it passes over a point on the earth's surface, there is a dramatic reverse in the wind direction. Hurricanes can also cause torrential rains which may result in floods and storm surges along the coastline (PAHO, 1992).

The U.S. National Weather Service has developed a computer model, SLOSH (Sea, Lake, and Overland Surges from Hurricanes), to be used for risk assessment of storm surges generated in hurricanes. The SLOSH model incorporates bathymetry and terrain information to determine inland flooding and water height over bays and estuaries. The parameters for input are track direction, landfall location, storm size, intensity, and forward speed. The model can be applied to either a segment of coastline or an island (U.S. National Report Committee, 1994).

Hurricane classification:

Hurricanes are often classified under the Saffir/Simpson scale, which gauges their wind speed and potential for damage. The following are the five categories of hurricanes recognized.

Category	Wind Speed		Damage Potential
	km/hr	mph	
HC1	119-151	74-95	Minimal
HC2	152-176	96-110	Moderate
HC3	177-209	111-130	Extensive
HC4	210-248	131-155	Extreme
HC5	over 248	over 155	Catastrophic

Local:

Pertaining to municipality, city or district as opposed to a larger territorial unit.

Post-traumatic Stress Disorder (PTSD):

PTSD is an anxiety disorder wherein one re-experiences severe traumatic stressors accompanied by increased avoidance and arousal symptoms associated with the trauma (*DSM-IV*, 1994).

Reaction:

Reaction has been defined as changes in behavior perceived by the survivors and brought about by the natural disaster.

Risk:

Given a hazardous situation, risk is the probability of expected losses (PAHO, 1992).

State:

Pertaining to one among many semi-autonomous political and territorial units forming a federated union.

Stress:

For the purpose of this manual, this term is defined as strain, pressure, or tension exerted upon an individual, a community, or a country. Therefore, the word is synonymous with tension.

Survivor:

For the purposes of this book, this term is defined as one who lived through a natural disaster, and is affected by it in some way.

Volcano:

According to the Random House Dictionary (1993), volcano is defined as a vent in the earth's crust through which lava, steam, ashes, expelled either continuously or at irregular intervals. Whereas there are 10,000 year-old active volcanoes in the Caribbean, currently, Mt. Soufriere in St. Vincent is the most active among them.

Volunteer:

One who freely chooses to serve others.

TEN LARGEST EARTHQUAKES IN THE WORLD
1900 to 1994

Table 5

Year	Month	Day	Time	Lat	Long	Location	Magnitude
1906	01	31	15:36:00.00	1.0 N	81.5 W	Ecuador	8.8 Mw
1922	11	11	04:32:36.00	28.5 S	70.0 W	Argentina	8.5 Mw
1938	02	01	19:04:18.00	5.25 S	130.5 E	Indonesia	8.5 Mw
1950	08	15	14:09:30.00	28.5 N	96.5 E	India	8.6 Mw
1952	11	04	16:58:26.00	52.75 N	159.9 E	Russia	9.0 Mw
1957	03	09	14:22:28.00	51.3 N	175.8 W	Alaska	9.1 Mw
1958	11	06	22:58:06.00	44.4 N	148.6 E	Japan (Kuril Islands)	8.7 Mw
1960	05	22	19:11:14.00	38.2 S	72.6 W	Chile	9.5 Mw
1964	03	28	03:36:14.00	61.1 N	147.5 W	Alaska	9.2 Mw
1965	02	04	05:01:22.00	51.3 N	178.6 E	Alaska	8.7 Mw

Prepared by the U.S. Geological Survey
National Earthquake Information Center

TYPES OF DISASTERS

1. Man-made disasters:

A. Planned and/or deliberate:

- Deforestation
- Fires (Arson)
- Massacres, genocides and holocausts
- Riots
- Terrorism
- Wars

B. Unplanned and/or accidental: Technical and/or chemical defects:

- Air, auto and rail accidents
- Collapses
- Explosions
- Fires
- Gas or chemical explosions
- Oil spills, and other contaminations

2. Natural disasters:

- Earthquakes
- Droughts and Pests
- Floods, Avalanches, and Mudslides
- Hurricanes, Tornado's and Tropical Cyclones
- Tsunamis (Tidal Waves)
- Volcanic eruptions

EFFECTS OF DISASTERS

Effects of natural disasters are multiple and can vary depending on the following variables:

- Natural hazard history of the area
- Type of the disaster
- Degree and severity of the impact
- Characteristics of the exposed elements
- Social, psychological, cultural, and spiritual resources available
- Response of the people effected by the disaster
- Response of others to the survivors' experiences

TYPES OF LOSSES

There are three types of losses: direct losses, indirect losses and undetected loses.

1. **Direct losses:** consist of resultant physical damage, such as victims who are killed or seriously injured as well as damage to the infrastructure of public services, damage to buildings, hospitals, industry, commerce, and a decrease in environmental safety.
2. **Indirect losses:** consist of the social and economic effects of a disaster. In the social arena, they may affect transportation, communication, public services and mass media. In the economic arena it may cause disruptions in commerce, construction, economy, trade, production, investment, import-export, tourism and development.
3. **Undetected losses:** are not identified at the time of the disaster or afterwards. These are losses difficult to calculate, measure, and/or value in terms dollars. These losses may include the loss of a community's positive image, loss of irreplaceable historical documents, loss of community cohesion, and loss of continuity and harmony.

PSYCHOLOGICAL PHASES OF DISASTERS

According to experts in disaster fields, five psychological phases are likely to occur after a disaster (*American Red Cross Manual on Disaster Health Services I*, 1992). These phases may vary in length and intensity depending upon vulnerability, extent of physical damage, and resources available.

1. *Initial impact phase*: characterized by increased anxiety and fears.
2. *Heroic phase*: characterized by survivors helping each other in efforts to deal with the catastrophe.
3. *Honeymoon phase*: characterized by experiences of joy at having survived and feeling important and special for receiving aid from various private and government organizations.
4. *Disillusionment phase*: characterized by increased frustration and resentment at officials and agencies for failing to provide assistance in a more timely fashion.
5. *Reconstitution phase*: characterized by thoughts and plans for reconstruction and acceptance of the need to assume responsibility for personal problems.

TYPES OF POSITIVE CHANGES

*There is occasions and causes why
and wherefore in all things.*

Shakespeare: King Henry V

Scientists, as well as health care professionals, generally focus on *only* the negative aspects of natural disasters. Notwithstanding the distinction, natural disasters present opportunities for growth, development, and improvement. According to Caplan (1964), proper and prompt intervention may not only lead an individual back to a pre-crisis state but to a higher level of mental health as well. Therefore, if the crisis resolution is successful, the individual learns new problem-solving behaviors and returns to a state of equilibrium, a steady state at a higher level of functioning than that which he experienced before the crisis occurred.

Positive Changes Post-Natural Disasters

1. Rebirthing experience
2. Rebuilding of communities destroyed or otherwise damaged
3. Developing newer and healthier coping skills
4. Adopting a new and more positive meaning in life
5. Helping one another in organized volunteer efforts
6. Taking steps toward prevention or reducing the impact of disaster
7. Experiencing existential growth

Numerous crisis theorists (Caplan, 1964; Gist and Stolz, 1982; Sime, 1980) have asserted that it is possible to increase one's resistance to mental disorders by helping that individual to extend his/her repertoire of effective problem-solving skills.

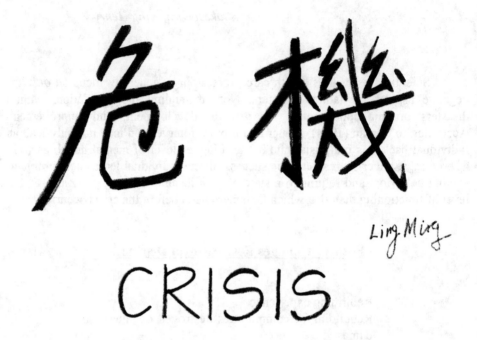

危機

Ling Ming

CRISIS

The Chinese characters representing the word crisis, indicated above, are a combination of the characters of danger and opportunity. Multiple losses affecting the individual post-disaster could be the danger, but learning from these loses and finding a positive meaning in them could be a challenge and an opportunity. According to Caplan's theory, crisis becomes an opportunity when intervention may occur properly, effectively, and promptly (Caplan, 1964). Therefore, the primary goal of the caregiver after a disaster is to provide high-level wellness, i.e., not only to restore the pre-disaster health status of the survivor, but to strive to surpass it.

Post-Natural Disaster Interventions:

- Enhancing the dynamic equilibrium between the individual and the environment through such intervention strategies as anticipatory guidance and ego strengthening, or general support.
- Evaluating the community's and the individual's histories in disaster management.
- Identifying the community's and the individual's habitual coping patterns and styles.
- Mobilizing the community's and the individual's internal and external resources.
- Lessening the effects of breakdown and maladaptation.

The United Nations Disaster Relief Organization (UNDRO)- currently United Nations Department for Humanitarian Affairs, together with the United Nations Educational, Scientific, and Cultural Organizations (UNESCO), sponsored a meeting of experts who proposed standardized definitions that have been widely accepted in the last few years. The 1994 report of this meeting, "Natural Disasters and Vulnerability Analysis," included the following definitions:

Hazard (**H**): The probability of occurrence of a potentially disastrous event during a certain period of time at a given site.

Vulnerability (**V**): the degree of loss of an element or group of elements at risk as a result of the probable occurrence of a disastrous event, expressed on a scale from 0 (no damage) to 1 (total loss).

Specific Risk (Rs): The degree of expected loss due to the occurrence of a specific event and as a function of the hazard and the vulnerability.

Elements at Risk (E): The people, buildings, public works, economic activities, utilities, public services and infrastructure exposed in a given area.

Total Risk (Rt): The death toll and number of wounded, property damage and impact on economic activity from the occurrence of a disastrous event.

Risk can be calculated in the following way:

Formula: RT = E (Elements at risk) • or X Rs (Specific risk) = E.(H.V.)

27

According to the Pan American Health Organization (PAHO, 1993, p. 5), once the hazard (Hi), understood as the probability that an event with an intensity greater than or equal to 'i' will take place during an exposure period 't' is known, and once vulnerability (Ve), understood as the intrinsic predisposition of an exposed element (e) to be affected by or to suffer a loss from the occurrence of an event with an intensity (i) is known, the risk (R_{ie}) can be understood as the probability that there will be a loss in the element (e) as a result of the occurrence of an event with an intensity greater than or equal to (i):

$$R_{ie} = (H_i, V_e)$$

PAHO further distinguishes between two concepts that mistakenly have been considered synonymous, but that are different both from the qualitative and quantitative points of view:

▶   The hazard or external risk factor of a subject or system that can occur at a specific site and at a given time, producing adverse effects on the individual system, the community, and/or the environment.

▶   The risk, damage, destruction, or expected loss derived from a combination of the probability of dangerous events and the vulnerability of the elements exposed to such threats.

An Overview of the Mental Health Outreach Program

The Mental Health Outreach Program (MHOP) was initially developed by the author following the 1988 earthquake in Armenia; parts of MHOP were replicated after the devastation wrought by Hurricane Andrew in Southern Florida, as well as following the 1994 earthquake in Southern California. For the purposes of MHOP, this author expands on the nursing process from its five phases into eight phases. The nursing process is a tool providing a systematic guideline for delivering care which includes assessment, diagnosis, planning, implementation and evaluation (Alfaro, 1986). Use of this modified version of the nursing process to intervene with national and international disaster problems has been very challenging for this author.

Eight Phases of the MHOP:

Preassessment

Assessment

Analysis

Community diagnosis

Planning

Implementation

Evaluation

Remodification

(Each of these MHOP Phases is presented in Chapters II through IX.)

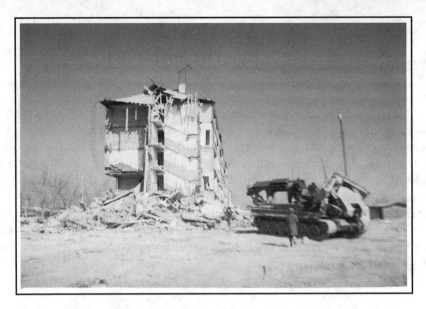

One month hence: A four story residential dwelling severely
damaged in Leninakan, Armenia
January, 1989

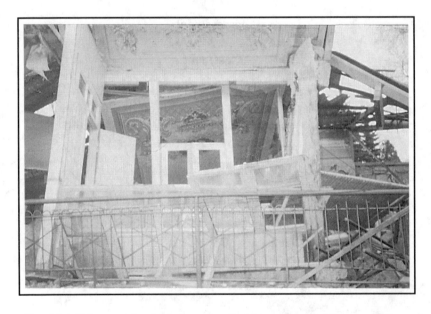

One month hence: A private one family home wrecked by the quake
in Spitak, Armenia
January, 1989

Photographs by: Dr. Anie Sanentz Kalayjian

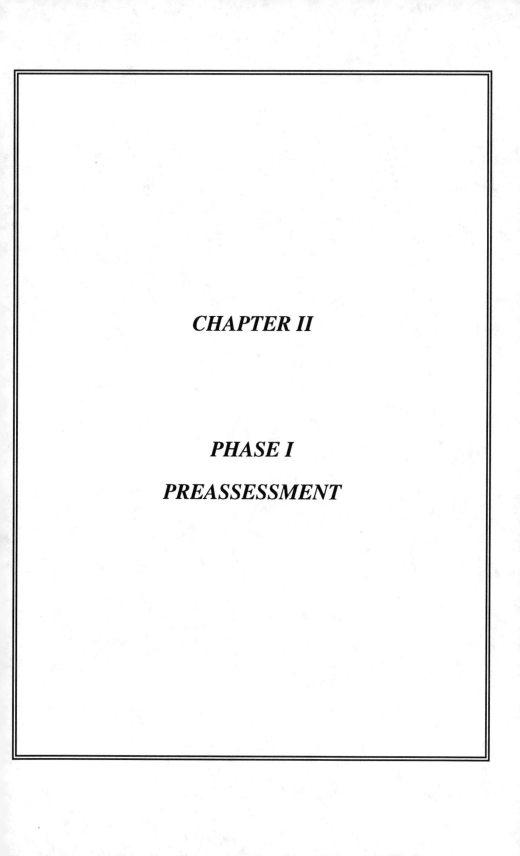

CHAPTER II

PHASE I

PREASSESSMENT

CHAPTER II

We shape our buildings,
and they shape us.

Winston Churchill

PHASE I

PREASSESSMENT

This phase occurs immediately prior to journeying to the disaster community. Ideally, preassessment begins immediately after the disaster and continues through the onset of the assessment phase. The following preassessment steps are necessary:

1. Familiarize oneself with the survivor community
2. Determine the physical extent of the damage
3. Determine the type of efforts made by others
4. Determine the needs as seen by other professionals
5. Communicate the program's goals
6. Prevent unnecessary duplication of effort
7. Delegate parts of the program to other professionals

Six Major Categories for Preassessment:

1. Survivor characteristics
2. Event Characteristics
3. Issues during the disaster relief
4. Pre- and post-disaster sociopolitical and economic climate
5. Resistance to change
6. Assessment instruments

The first two categories are adopted from Bolin's (1985) categories for assessment. The last four categories are based on the author's professional experience in disaster management. A discussion of these six categories follows.

1. Survivor Characteristics

To learn about the survivor community, one needs to research recent media, speak with people familiar with that community, as well as with people originally from that community. The following are some of the questions to ask:

1. What are the geographic size and characteristics of the community?
2. What are the ethnic backgrounds or nationalities of the residents?
3. What are their religious/spiritual beliefs?
4. What is their economic situation?
5. What are the languages spoken?
6. What are the resources available to them, individually and collectively?
7. What are their previous disaster experiences?
8. What are their views regarding receiving assistance from outside of their community?
9. Does the community have insurance available to them for natural catastrophes?
10. What percentage of the community may have purchased insurance?

Also recommended is the collection of information pertaining to the history of the disaster in the region.

Research the following areas:

1. History of natural disasters, including floods, earthquakes, mudslides or any other such recorded events.
2. Date of most recent natural disaster.
3. Types of complications causing further physical deterioration after the last disaster, such as aftershocks, fires or mudslides, etc.
4. Number of people affected during the last disaster.
5. Strengths and resources exhibited by the people during the last disaster.
6. Difficulties and deficits exhibited by the people after the last disaster.

Survivor Characteristics in Armenia

Who were the survivors of the 1988 earthquake in Armenia? They were intelligent, hard-working, peaceful, religious, family-oriented, and hospitable people (Jordon, 1978). The Republic of Armenia is geographically the smallest of the former Soviet Republics, with a population of approximately four million, and is the most entrepreneurial and economically fastest-growing republic (Walker, 1991). The historical record shows an Armenian presence in the general region of

Asia Minor and the Caucasus dating back over three millennia (Ishkhanian, 1989). Its history through the centuries is one of enduring oppression, war, relocation and survival. From the end of the fourteenth century until 1991, Armenia had only two years of independence (1918-1920), yet its people, culture and language have survived. On September 23, 1991, Armenia once again declared independence. For the first time in 71 years, the Armenian people freely elected a President and Representatives to the Republic's Parliament, the Supreme Soviet, from a slate of candidates representing a variety of political movements and organizations.

In discussing their history, Armenians mention three things. First, they mention their religion. This is a point of great pride since Armenia became the first nation to adopt Christianity in 301 AD as its national religion. Second, they mention their language. The Armenian language is a distinct branch of the Indo-European family of languages, with a unique thirty-eight character alphabet. Lastly, they mention their survival of the Ottoman-Turkish Genocide. From 1895 to 1923, the Armenian Nation was brought to the brink of annihilation as almost two million Armenians, more than half the Armenian population, were massacred by the Ottoman Turkish rulers. To this day, the Genocide is denied by the current Turkish government. This denial causes tremendous feelings of anger and resentment, with no reparation or resolution (Kalayjian, et al. 1991a). During World War II, and for over seventy years under Communism, Armenians experienced yet more pain and suffering. This was a system that relied on oppression of individual needs for the sake of the party and any rebellious gesture could lead to one's disappearance. Pain and suffering continued on in the post-independence era, due to territorial conflict within Azerbaijan over Nagorno-Karabagh. Adding to the suffering has been the Azeri blockade of Armenia which began in 1988 and as of 1995, is yet to be lifted.

The literacy rate is comparatively high in Armenia as virtually all Armenian children attend school for 8 to 10 years from age 6 to 16.

People are industrious yet poor as the economy has been decimated by decades of Soviet rule, further exacerbated by the Azeri blockade.

As in many third world countries, an insurance industry is non-existent. As per the Soviet design, health care is free in Armenia, but the quality and availability vary greatly.

Summary of Survivor Characteristics in Armenia:

1. Smallest geographical republic in the former Soviet Union.
2. Population: Four million.
3. Historical presence: Over three millennia.
4. Religion: First Christian Nation, 301 AD.
5. Language: Indo-European, 38-character alphabet.

6. Education: High literacy.
7. Economy: Industrious yet poor.
8. Survival: 1895-1923 Ottoman Turkish Genocide of the Armenians, two million massacred.
9. Conflict with Turkey due to denial of Genocide.
10. Conflict with Azerbaijan over Nagorno-Karabagh.
11. Azeri blockade of Armenia.
12. Struggling for democracy.
13. Insurance: None exists.

Survivor Characteristics in Southern Florida:

According to the 1995 *Information Please Almanac*, Florida is one of the nation's fastest growing states. Its population has grown from 2.8 million in 1950 to over 13.7 million in 1993. Florida's top industry is tourism (in 1992 the state entertained more than 40 million visitors from all over the world). Other industries include agriculture, manufacturing and international trade.

Florida's residential population is 83.1% white, 13.6% African American, 0.3% Native American, 1.2% Asian, and 1.8% other races. Hispanics may belong to any of the above racial groups. A majority of the Hispanic residents (62.5%) live in the southern part of the state. Although survivors were mostly Americans, there were a large number of legal and illegal residents from Cuba, Haiti, Jamaica, and Mexico.

Miami, located in southern Florida, is the second largest city in the state. Miami experienced one of its most monumental population booms during the 1960's, when about 260,000 Cuban refugees arrived seeking freedom.

Florida ranks fourth in the U.S. in public education enrollment and 29th in expenditures per pupil. Of its population, 79.6% will complete four years of high school or more, and 19.8% four years of college or more (*The Universal Almanac*, 1995).

Florida's gross state product, as of 1990, was $244.62 billion, placing it sixth in the nation, ahead of most small nations.

Hurricane Andrew struck a wide area, and impacted a community of varying socioeconomic levels. Some survivors who had resided in Homestead for over thirty years had experienced another devastating hurricane in 1965. Though there was a lack of coherence and community homogeneity as a whole, there were several pockets of cohesion. These included senior citizens, illegal immigrants, legal immigrants, the armed forces and recently relocated families from the Northern and Western parts of the country.

Various homeowner's insurance policies were available to residents. However, although many residents purchased insurance, not all obtained special hurricane or flood insurance.

Summary of Survivor Characteristics in Southern Florida:

1. Fastest growing state.
2. Population: 13.7 million.
3. Religion: Catholic majority.
4. Education: 79.6% graduate from high school.
5. Economy: Gross state product $244.62 billion.
6. Many young communities unfamiliar with hurricanes.
7. Pockets of a variety of ethnic communities not inter-related.
8. Many residential communities for the older population.
9. Many tourists from Canada, Europe and other parts of the United States.
10. Air Force Base community.
11. Migrant farm workers in trailer parks.
12. Sailors and other residents in boat houses.
13. Survivors were from all socioeconomic levels.
14. Insurance: Available, but not all were insured.

Survivor Characteristics in California:

Searching through the *New York Times* and other newspapers to gather information regarding survivor characteristics in Southern Los Angeles was futile. Using CD-ROM, the author printed 58 abstracts dating from January 17 to February 21, 1994, and found 99% of the articles addressed the event characteristics while none addressed survivor characteristics.

In 1993 the population of California stood at 31,210,750, making it the most populous state in the U.S. The racial composition as of 1990 was 69% white, 7.4% African American, 0.8% Native American, 9.6% Asian, and 13.2% other races. Hispanic Americans are 25.8% of the population (*The Universal Almanac*, 1995).

As of 1990, the gross state product was $744.73 billion, ranking California first in the nation.

In 1990, Los Angeles, in southern California, had a population of 3,485,398, making it the second largest city - - after New York - - in the U.S. (*The Universal Almanac*, 1995).

Public education enrollment was 5,285,000 in 1993, ranking California first in the nation. Per pupil expenditure was $4,584, placing it 35th in the U.S. Of the student population, 79.7% attain four years of high school or more, and 25% four years of college or more (*The Universal Almanac*, 1995).

Los Angelinos contend daily with smog, auto accidents and traffic jams. Through their history, Los Angelinos have also experienced a variety of natural disasters, such as mudslides, fires, earthquakes, and floods. The metropolis lies on the San Andres Fault, which comprises fractures in the crest of the earth along California's coast line and down the Gulf of California.

Various home owner's insurance policies were available to the residents. The majority of residents were insured for earthquakes.

Survivors of the Los Angeles earthquake of January 17, 1994 were long-term residents of the area, with the exception of the student population of the University of California-Northridge. A large number of survivors were well-prepared and informed regarding earthquakes.

Summary of Survivor Characteristics in California:

1. Population: As of 1993 - 31,210, 750
2. Education: Public education enrollment taking first in the nation.
3. Economy: As of 1990, $744.73 Billion gross state product.
4. Religion: Mostly Christian, but mixed
5. Survivors: Largely white American, long-term residents of the area.
6. Small number of legal residents from Armenia fled the 1988 quake.
7. Small number of Mexican and African-Americans.
8. Largely established communities who have experienced earthquakes.
9. Area with most damage was Northridge, where there was a large student population from all around the U.S.
10. Survivors were from all socioeconomic levels.
11. Insurance: Most were insured.

2. Event Characteristics

The next area of assessment is centered on the event characteristics. The following are the ten questions to ask:

1. What is the extent of the physical damage?
2. What is the extent of casualties?
3. To what extent has the community been destroyed?
4. To what extent has the community's infrastructure been destroyed?
5. What percentage of the population required evacuation and to where has it been evacuated?
6. What is the effect on housing?

36

7. What is the geographic area affected?
8. What percentage of the survivors have lost work?
9. What is the impact on hospitals?
10. To what extent have the transportation and communications systems been affected?

Event Characteristics in Armenia:

On Wednesday, December 7, 1988, at 11:41 AM, a devastating earthquake shook the Republic of Armenia (Soviet Armenia) for 40 seconds. This catastrophic destruction occurred in a zone where several plates of the earth's surface converge, which occasionally results in devastating consequences when movement occurs. Although the quake did not come as a total surprise to American and Soviet experts in the field, according to Purkaru of the geological institute in Frankfurt (Sullivan, 1988), due to gross unpreparedness and lack of emergency and evacuation plans, the community experienced the quake as a total nightmare. "If there was a horror movie like the quake, I would have not believed it," stated Gurgen, a 32-year old survivor from Leninakan (now Gumri

In 893 AD, a quake in the same general area of Armenia caused 20,000 deaths. In 1667, another earthquake in that general region had claimed 80,000 lives and in the late 1800's, yet another devastating quake had taken place there. "I have Chernobyl behind me, but I have never seen anything like this," Yevgeny I. Chazov, the Soviet Health Minister, told the government newspaper Izvestia after visiting the scene with fellow physicians (Fein, 1988).

Measuring 6.9 on the Richter scale, the quake occurred in an area highly vulnerable to seismic activity. It destroyed two-thirds of Leninakan, Armenia's second-largest city (now Vanatzor, population about 30,000), half of Kirovakan (population 150,000), obliterated Spitak - the epicenter (a town of about 30,000), and heavily damaged some fifty-six of 150 villages and towns in the northwest corner of Armenia, near the Turkish border. Initial reports of casualties spoke of "thousands" which soon became "tens of thousands" and went on to climb day-by-day to 130,000, even though the official death toll was announced as 25,000. In the end, there were about 500,000 people handicapped, approximately 500,000 children orphaned, and over half-a-million, one sixth of Armenia's population, left homeless. The exact number of human loss was very difficult to determine for several reasons: the uncertain number of refugees from the February 1988 massacres in the Azerbaijani cities of Baku and Sumgait, the poor record-keeping procedures, and, finally, the Soviet government's covert style of operations. Therefore, the above estimates, or any estimates from this incident, are only provisional. Proportional losses in the United States would have amounted to six million dead and 40 million homeless. The physical damage was estimated at $20 billion (U.S.).

Unlike other earthquakes, where there is often a prediction of occurrence, this event was largely unanticipated by the surviving community. It impacted a very large segment of the local population and caused tremendous property damage. All hospitals, schools, churches and community centers were severely damaged or destroyed, unlike the Mexican quake of 1986, the San Francisco quake of 1989, and the Los Angeles quake of 1994. Survivors were forced to head for the capital, Yerevan, to receive emergency medical care. This meant traveling four to six hours, instead of the usual two hours, in extremely crowded conditions and on roads that were partially destroyed by the quake. Therefore, the delay caused additional casualties. "My only brother, ten years old, died in my arms in the car going to Yerevan," stated Nayiri, a sixteen year old female Armenian survivor from Spitak. In the earthquake region, survivors had no areas left intact in their community through which to seek support. In turn, this made relocation a necessity and created additional stress and trauma. Further trauma was caused by the Soviet government when it decided to relocate women and children to Yerevan and other Soviet Republics, while keeping the men in the earthquake zone to help "clean up." According to Terr (1989), families cope better if they remain together after a trauma. Therefore, these relocations and separations further aggravated the trauma by shattering and displacing family units.

Assistance from all over the world poured into Armenia. Within the first ten days, $50,000,000 worth of goods, food and supplies were delivered to Yerevan's airport from around the world, overwhelming the damaged distribution system. This airlift marked the first time since World War II that the Soviet government had accepted disaster assistance from the United States. In all, the American government spent about four million U.S. dollars, and U.S. Air Force and National Guard planes were used to fly in the relief supplies. Private contributions from Americans in the first four weeks following the earthquake reached about 34 million dollars. The grand total given by all countries outside the Soviet Union reached 106 million dollars (Simon, 1989). According to U.S. Senator Simon, in view of the fact that the United States represents 20 percent of the world's economy, what the US did as a nation was not that impressive. However, aid sent by the US government to the Soviet Union and its acceptance was unprecedented. When the Marshall Plan was announced in 1948, the Soviets would accept no American aid whatsoever. Therefore, the fact that aid was given and received was a healthy sign (Simon, 1989).

Summary of Event Characteristics in Armenia

1. No prediction.

2. Impacted a very large geographical segment, two of the largest cities, and 56 villages.
3. No intact community centers.
4. No intact hospitals.
5. Infrastructure damage. (e.g., streets, bridges, etc.)
6. Relocation policies of the Soviet government.
7. Very large segment of the population relocated, with no accurate records kept.
8. Over 500,000 homeless, handicapped or otherwise affected.
9. Over 75,000 dead/missing.
10. Over $20 billion in damages.
11. No electricity, running water, gas or telephone service for over 6 months.
12. No emergency or evacuation plans.
13. No earthquake preparedness.

Event Characteristics in Southern Florida:

A ferocious hurricane slammed into the Bahamas Sunday afternoon on August 23, 1992, with 120 mph winds, heavy rain and a surging tide. Four people were reported dead as a result of the storm. The damage in Louisiana, in the north west, while severe in places, did not compare with the panorama of ruin in Southern Florida. Officials reported that the storm left over 250,000 Floridians homeless. As it ended its journey across the Gulf of Mexico, Hurricane Andrew struck as far west as the major populated areas around New Orleans, moving inland over sparsely populated marshlands, and doing its worst damage in small towns along Interstate 90 from Morgan City to New Iberia. The marshes and the swamps took the brunt of the storm in Louisiana, thus causing less human loss there.

By 2 AM on Sunday, August 23, 1992, the eye of the storm was about 60 miles from Florida, moving westward at 18 mph with wind speeds of nearly 140 mph. By 1:30 AM of the same morning, high winds in advance of the storm toppled trees and knocked out electrical transformers in the Miami Beach area and sunk boats in Biscayne Bay. The eye of the storm passed south of Miami, between Homestead and Cutler Ridge, which meant that the strongest winds struck the Homestead, Cutler Ridge, and Coconut Grove areas. The strong east-to-west winds pushed the hurricane along a bit faster than might otherwise have been the case, causing it to clear Florida in a relatively brief three hours. This was a category 4 storm on the Saffir-Simpson scale of hurricane intensity, where category 5 is the strongest. The course of this storm appeared to be following closely that of Hurricane Betsy in 1965, a Category 3 storm that struck both

Southern Florida and New Orleans, causing $1.5 billion worth of damage and killing 75 people.

Residents of Dade County, which includes Miami Beach, Key Biscayne, Fort Lauderdale, Homestead and other low-lying coastal areas, were urged by authorities to evacuate. Floridians underestimated the damage that such a storm can cause, and did not adhere to the official orders. Thus, their history did not serve them well. Those who had lived in Florida all their lives did not abide by the evacuation orders. Some responded by saying "We trust Mother Nature," and some others - "It can't be that bad, we're going to ride it out," and yet others - "You've got to die sometime. It can't be *that* bad." Many people organized hurricane parties and bought cases of beer, chips and cigarettes to celebrate, some in denial and some to numb the pain of the impact.

It seemed some individuals were lulled by the hope that Andrew would turn northward at the last minute toward Georgia and the Carolinas, as Hurricane Hugo did in 1989, and as several other storms have done in recent years. But a high-pressure system extending east from Jacksonville kept that from occurring and pushed the storm westward. On Sunday, August 23, 1994, the National Hurricane Center declared a hurricane watch from Titusville, near Cape Canaveral, Florida to Key West and a hurricane warning for the area from Vero Beach south through the Florida Keys.

The evacuation orders, which began Sunday morning, covered a 200-mile belt from Key West to Fort Lauderdale, east of the main coastal highways, US Route 1 and Interstate 95. They extended to low-lying areas and to mobile-home communities further north, and to areas along the southwestern coast as well. One million people were told to evacuate. In Dade County, which includes Miami, 70,000 people spent the night in 48 shelters set up in churches and schools. At 7:30 PM the same night a Dade County official stated at a news conference that they could no longer provide any special evacuation assistance to those who may have needed it, as they had exhausted their resources. In Broward County, north of Miami, 21,000 people had gone to public shelters by midnight. Miami International Airport was closed by 9:30 PM on Sunday, leaving travelers stranded at the airport.

In Key West, many tourists who had been unable to leave on commercial or chartered flights tried to hire taxis to drive them to Miami, 164 miles to the northeast, but their attempts were in vain. On that Sunday evening, most of the Southern Florida gas stations, hardware stores, pharmacies and groceries that had been mobbed with customers since midnight on Saturday were closed. The few stores that did remain open did not have such essentials as water, flashlight batteries, canned goods or bread. In hardware stores, people were waiting in line for hours to buy sheets of plywood to board up their windows. Plywood prices originally quoted at around $22 per sheet had increased to $40.

On August 24, 1994, several thousand National Guard troops were sent in to join local law enforcement officers who were trying to prevent looting, which was reported throughout the day in the hurricane-devastated area. Miami and Dade County, the jurisdiction that surrounds the city, imposed a curfew from late evening to early morning to prevent looting. The Air Force had evacuated all but 18 of its 4,300 military personnel from its base at Homestead over the weekend, and most of its F-16 fighter jets and C-130 transports had been sent to bases in South Carolina and Georgia.

Main roads, especially U.S. Route 1, as well as side streets, were filled with debris, parts of roofs, sailboats, other pieces of furniture and palm trees yanked out of the ground with balls of roots and turf still attached. Some people returning later could not even find their streets. The roads were further jammed due to residents who had evacuated the area the day before, and who were now returning to their homes. Small airplanes were strewn along runways at the Tamiami Airport, and the hangars that had sheltered them had been blown away. Street signs were blown off their designated poles, creating yet additional problems for drivers, as well as residents. There was the overall absence of basic public services, such as water, electricity, gas and telephones.

At the South Miami Hospital in Homestead, the generator failed and there was no running water or telephones. Staff had to work day and night to help the injured and evacuate patients to a nearby hospital. One man described the situation by saying, "I spent two years in Vietnam and I have not seen anything like this." In some areas extensive looting took place. Therefore, there were strictly enforced curfews, helicopters patrolling overhead, heaps of rubble, tent cities and overturned cars.

Other related losses also occurred, such as the crash of a small plane carrying aid to the victims of Hurricane Andrew. The plane crashed into the roof of a house in Miramar near Miami. Two people died in the crash, and another was seriously injured.

After a five day journey of destruction, Hurricane Andrew ripped through the oil towns and Cajun country of Southern Louisiana on August 26, 1994.

Summary of Event Characteristics in Southern Florida:

1. A category 4 storm, the most powerful hurricane in about 30 years to hit Florida.
2. Predicted about 48 hours before the hurricane struck.
3. Hurricane warning was made.
4. Winds as high as 140 miles an hour.
5. Slammed into a 200-mile belt from Key West to Fort Lauderdale.
6. Hit Bahamas and moved toward Florida in less than 24 hours.

7. Over 750,000 people evacuated.
8. Over 250,000 people displaced.
9. 100,000 residents left South Dade County (about 27% of the total).
10. 180.00 people left homeless.
11. 15 people dead in Florida (a total of 52 hurricane-related deaths in Florida, Louisiana and the Bahamas combined).
12. $30 billion in property damages.
13. 8,373 single-family homes destroyed; 37245 had major damage and 40,632 had minor damage.
14. 8,974 mobile homes destroyed, 1,100 had major damage and 519 had minor damage.
15. Nine public schools destroyed and 23 had heavy damage.
16. 2,100 traffic signal lights damaged.
17. 50,000 trees destroyed in Dade County parks.
18. 33% of coral reefs damaged at Biscayne National Park.
19. 90% of South Dade's native pinelands, tropical hardwood hammocks and mangroves destroyed or damaged.
20. 32,900 acres of farmland damaged.
21. 300,000 jobs lost.
22. 8,000 businesses destroyed or damaged.
23. $18 billion estimated insurance loss.
24. 4,082 complaints of fraud were filed against contractors, licensed and unlicensed.

Event Characteristics in Southern California:

Southern California's January 17, 1994, 4 AM earthquake measured 6.8 on the Richter Scale, damaging thousands of buildings in densely populated Los Angeles and Ventura Counties, killing 57, and injuring 7,300 people. This quake involved movement along a blind thrust fault. The "big one" Californians have been promised for years will be no blind thrust. Instead, like the 1906 San Francisco quake, it is expected that it will be the work of the San Andreas Fault. The 1994 quake was described as having erratic behavior. The tumbler wrecked one building while sparing a near-by twin and caused hundreds of millions of dollars in damages miles from the epicenter, while sparing buildings that were much closer. Parking garages also faired poorly, perhaps as a result of pounding caused by unusually large vertical accelerations (Rosenbaum and McManamy, 1994).

According to the preliminary estimates by the Los Angeles Fire Department, there were 200 buildings with major damage; the quake was especially devastating to buildings with fewer than six stories, and left 600 buildings with moderate damage. There was extensive damage to concrete tilt-up buildings used for light industry and wood-frame, concrete-block and older concrete-frame structures typically built in the 1970's. The most severe damage involved shopping malls, parking structures, concrete tilt-up buildings and residential apartments. Total damage estimates kept climbing.

There was major infrastructure damage which occurred at two curvilinear elevated ramps leading from the Antelope Valley Freeway to the Golden State Freeway. One span collapsed from the southbound Route 14 connector to northbound I-5 and three collapsed from the southbound 14 to southbound I-5 (Rosenbaum and Post, 1994). The California Department of Transportation (Caltrans) was confident that within a year they would be able to repair the four destroyed locations. Jim Roberts, Caltrans Deputy Director of Transportation Engineering, estimated the cost of replacing the structures at $100 million, the maximum sum the Federal Highway Administration (FHA) can authorize as emergency relief. Designing the freeway repair began on the day of the earthquake by FHA staff and consultants. FHA expected to use parts of the original drawings as the superstructures would remain more or less the same (Green 1994).

Commercial property losses were also severe. Among the companies forced to relocate post-quake was Packard Bell Electronics. GTE's customer service office in Granada Hills was condemned and Pacific Bell suffered $25 million in property damage from the quake and its subsequent aftershocks. The United Parcel Service sorting facility in San Fernando suffered a collapsed roof causing severe damage. All of Tandy Corporations' Los Angeles area retail outlets sustained damage ranging from mild to severe. Additionally, the Los Angeles entertainment industry was also sent reeling by the quake (Wojcik, 1994).

Health care providers in Southern California were fearful of losing both their physicians and their patients. Cigna Healthcare of Southern California was forced to close 2 of its 28 outpatient health care centers in Canoga Park and Granada Hills since both were located near the quake's epicenter in the Northridge-Reseda area of the San Fernando Valley. Some 34 hospital buildings and medical offices sustained damage from the powerful quake (de Lafuente, 1994).

Oil and gas facilities in the Los Angeles area suffered only minor losses. Los Angeles area refineries withstood the shock fairly well, but damage was reported at one gasoline distribution facility. Meanwhile, ARCO's Line 1, which carries crude oil from the San Joaquim Valley to the company's refinery near Long Beach - - a city in south western California, south of Los Angeles - - suffered at least four ruptures in the San Fernando and Santa Clarita Valleys near Pyramid Lake in the Coast Range mountains. The most serious break allowed an estimated 2,900 to 3,000 gallons of oil to leak from the line into a 12-mile stretch of the Santa Clara River near Newhall, about 12 miles north of the epicenter. ARCO estimated the cleanup would take about one month, and the line was out of operation for 3 to 4 weeks post-quake.

Summary of Event Characteristics in Southern California:

1. No prediction or warning.
2. Severe infrastructure damage.
3. Oil leak.
4. Erratic behavior of the quake,
5. Unusual pounding due to unusually large vertical accelerations.
6. Especially devastating to buildings with fewer than 6 stories.
7. 1.1 million lost electrical power as well as gas service.
8. 3,500 aftershocks.
9. 34 hospital buildings and medical offices were damaged.
10. $30 billion in damages.
11. Killed 61 people.
12. Injured 7,300 people.
13. Californians thought it was "The Big One."

3. Issues During Disaster Relief

When disaster strikes, scientists and seismologists tend to talk about it as if it occurred in a vacuum. The media also has a distinct tendency to dissect the disaster out of the everyday issues of the surviving community. The following are some of the questions to ask when attempting to assess the issues during a disaster:

1. What is the community response to the disaster?
2. What is the national response to the disaster?
3. What is the international response to the disaster?
4. What is the evacuation process like?
5. What is the extent of assistance to the surviving community?
6. Is the assistance reaching the survivors in an organized manner?
7. Are there any political or economic issues which could affect progress?
8. Are there volunteer organizations within the surviving community?
9. Are the channels of communication open and clear?
10. Is there community cohesion and harmony?

In Armenia:

The disaster response was somewhat different in Armenia compared to that seen in Florida and California. Overwhelming international attention was received due to the interruption of President Gorbachev's visit to the United States. But this did not result in an organized rescue effort. Efforts were extremely disorganized, began too late and resulted in chaos. The warning system was out-dated, old-fashioned or just dysfunctional, and the rescue equipment was either broken or insufficient.

Though assistance poured in from all around the world, Armenia's airport was not equipped to deal with that volume and therefore, many planes could not land. The planes that were able to land just unloaded their goods on the runway. Much of the other assistance that went through Moscow did not make it to Armenia in its entirety. This lasted until Armenian voluntary organizations took over the distribution and management of the funds, as well as the goods.

In Southern Florida:

Hurricane Andrew caught the community by surprise. Although some people were prepared - - having bought batteries, groceries, bottled water and plywood to board up their windows - - most people had not taken the threat of the storm seriously. The majority reacted by saying, "We've been hearing these threats every year; nothing is going to happen; I am sure we'll deal with this," and "Not me, I think this one will blow over us. This area hasn't been hit in a long time." These attitudes, borne of familiarity and disbelief, led to greater shock immediately following the hurricane. Many members of the community intended to ride out the storm no matter what anyone said. Although the author was not there during the initial disaster relief, she was able to follow the relief process by way of radio and television announcements. Many survivors stated that this had been the closest that they had ever come to death. The community reacted with overwhelming fear and uncertainty.

Red Cross volunteer forces began to intervene immediately with shelters in churches, schools and other community outreach centers. Other volunteer groups, including church groups, were organized to assist the surviving community.

Hospitals in the area, especially SMH Homestead Hospital and South Miami Hospital, were treating survivors around the clock. SMH Homestead Hospital displayed a sign over the doorway to its emergency room that read, "We beat Andrew like nobody else could." Professional nurses, psychologists and other staff donated their time and expertise to help those in need. Although SMH Homestead Hospital itself sustained $2 million in damages and had to close for five days to repair, clean, stock and restore utilities, most of the employees worked nonstop. Some of the employees did not come back; they chose to relocate. One nursing unit at SMH Homestead Hospital lost over 50% of its staff. Fortunately, volunteers and traveling nurses from across the nation arrived to fill in where necessary.

The Federal Emergency Management Agency (FEMA) was also visible some time later. Although initially FEMA received criticism for being late, they were effective in providing travel trailers to qualified applicants - - often to families of five or six.

On Friday, August 28, 1992, four days after the hurricane, Pentagon officials announced that 5,000 troops were being sent from Fort Bragg in Fayetteville, NC, along with portable kitchens, medicine, supplies, helicopters and bulldozers. They set up tents for shelter and kitchens to feed 6,000 people three meals a day. Nevertheless a professional disaster relief specialist characterized this response as "modest and tardy."

On Monday August 24, 1992, the Medical Examiner's Office, which is equipped to handle an average of 10 deaths a day, had to deal with 66 bodies. Offices of Emergency Management were also overwhelmed. Ms. Kate Hale, director of Dade County's Office of Emergency Management, announced on Sunday night before the hurricane that the resources of her office had been completely exhausted and that they would no longer be able to provide special evacuation assistance to those in need. By midnight Sunday, 21,000 people had gone to public shelters in Broward County, north of Miami. Some shelters were packed to twice their capacity, and county officials had asked for emergency donations of food.

On August 27, 1992 Dade County officials directed the County Attorney to file a Federal Lawsuit in an effort to postpone a statewide primary election scheduled for Tuesday, on the grounds that extensive hurricane damage would not allow Dade County voters access the polls.

Other calamities also occurred during the relief. Two people were killed and another injured as a small plane carrying aid to the victims of the hurricane crashed onto the roof of a house in Miramar, near Miami.

Channels of communication were disrupted; there were no telephones, electricity or mail. Community members tried to deal with this chaotic state by staying with friends, neighbors or at places of work.

In Southern California:

Unlike the community in Southern Florida, the community in southern California did not have pre-warning or time for preparation before the earthquake. Although earthquakes occur frequently in Southern California, the magnitude of this Valley earthquake caught the community by surprise.

The evacuation process was organized and systematic. Survivors were able to find shelters in the vicinity with no difficulty.

National response, through FEMA and the ARC, was swift, expeditious and prompt. Both FEMA and ARC set up clinics throughout the hardest hit areas of southern California immediately after the earthquake. Professional nurses and mental health professionals volunteered to help through the above-mentioned organizations.

As early as one month after the earthquake, many of the FEMA disaster assistance centers had been closed. Hospitals and community centers were providing primary care and counseling. Much of the damage had been cleaned up. Survivors were suffering from post-traumatic stress and minor acute illnesses, such as colds and the flu. Some survivors had Valley Fever, a fungal infection of the respiratory system. People contracted the ailment from spores that were released from the earth by the quake and were inhaled from the huge cloud of dust that hung over the area during the hours following the disaster.

Eight collapsed segments of the freeway system caused massive traffic jams. Exasperated commuters resorted to what would have been unthinkable in their car-freeway-worship culture: they began using commuter trains. Metrolink, the city's embryonic light-rail system, reported a tripling of morning passengers from 10,000 to 30,000 on its four lines. Even after freeway detours were eliminated, Metrolink maintained 70% of the new ridership.

Although President Clinton quickly asked Congress for $6.6 billion in disaster relief, State leaders moved with less alacrity. State Assembly Speaker Willie Brown took more than a week to propose a one-year half-cent sales tax increase to raise $1.5 billion for earthquake relief. The U.S. Department of Transportation released $50 million for emergency work and the City of Los Angeles cut bureaucratic red tape and helped expedite the selection of construction managers for demolition and debris cleanup.

In addition to the assistance of federal, national and voluntary organizations, other agencies, especially corporations and a number of advertising agencies in Los Angeles, launched collection drives to help employees who sustained damage or losses in the devastating earthquake, hoping to ease recovery amid the mental and physical aftershocks plaguing the region.

4. Pre- and Post-Disaster Sociopolitical and Economic Climate

An examination of the pre-disaster sociopolitical and economic climate, as it influences the resources available to the survivor community, is an essential step within the preassessment phase of the plan.

Armenia:

During the ten months preceding the quake, Armenia was experiencing sociopolitical tension and was economically drained. This was due to the conflict with neighboring Azerbaijan over Nagorno-Karabagh, a 4,000 square kilometer enclave mostly populated by Armenians and locally ruled by Armenians until 1923, when Josef Stalin gave it to Soviet Azerbaijan. In early 1988, Armenia challenged Gorbachev and put "Glasnost" and "Perestroika" to their first true test, but failed. As a result, over 200,000 Armenian refugees from Azerbaijan came to already overcrowded Armenia. In February 1988, there was yet another massacre in Sumgait, Azerbaijan, where dozens of Armenians were killed, houses were burned and women were raped and set on fire (Kalayjian, 1991b). Noteworthy is that seismologists described the quake area as a "structural knot," engendered by the interaction of several rigid plates (Sullivan, 1988). Ironically, this paralleled the sociopolitical and emotional situation: political agitation, tension, anger, resentment, disappointment and mistrust, due, at least partly, to rigid attitudes.

Southern Florida:

Before Hurricane Andrew, both politically and economically, the community was in a state of equilibrium. After the hurricane, though, there was a tremendous problem caused by the migrant construction workers who traveled from South Carolina, Georgia, Alabama, even from as far away as Michigan and New Jersey, to make a "quick buck." They lived in roadside camps with their shotguns and 9-mm pistols, drugs and drinks. In one incident, a roofer was stabbed 100 times and in another, soldiers who patrolled the area reported seeing a roofer bite off another man's ear and then spit it out. Local Police Officers referred to them as "roofers from hell." The wife of a roofer from Indiana said, "The price of one's life is less than a 12 pack of beer." According to Cathy Booth, a survivor in Key Largo (1993), one carpenter from Pennsylvania was living in his aging Scout van at "Camp Mad Max" because he couldn't afford a hotel. Thieves had taken his car battery, radio, tools and even his Penn State floor mats. His body was covered with infected mosquito bites, and on his back, an antibiotic cream covered a patch of ringworm. He was planning to cure it himself by sanding down the skin and then washing it with Clorox.

The author met several survivors who complained about the roofers and the construction people. One survivor said that she had gone through eight different construction companies in less than two months. Mary, a registered nurse from the S M H - Homestead, said that the first contractor took the deposit and never returned, the second contractor came and promised to return the next day and never did and the third one came to give the estimate and began drinking an alcoholic beverage. Mary then fired the third contractor, but in the meantime, she had already taken three days off from work, with no compensation and no contractor, while still living in a trailer.

Southern California:

The socioeconomic status of California had been somewhat depressed for several years before the earthquake of January 17, 1994. The real estate market had been depressed and Californians were hoping for change.

Many builders and construction personnel interviewed by this author had complained about the economic situation. Political, racial and ethnic tensions prevailed. Approximately one year before the quake, fear and uncertainty had permeated the state following the 1992 riots of Southern Los Angeles due to the racially sensitive Rodney King trial verdict, which had led to the destruction of many stores, cars and houses. Three days of looting and rioting rocked the city in reaction to the jury acquittal of white police officers who had been videotaped as they beat Rodney King, an African-American motorist.

5. Resistance to Change

Whenever faced with an unplanned change, community leaders/mental health professionals need to consider the resistance to this change, how to mobilize the community and how to utilize this resistance to benefit the people. The Mental Health Outreach Program (MHOP) to Armenia was a challenge for this author, an American-Armenian mental health professional. The most difficult challenge of all was to gaining access to the Soviet Union in order to organize and deliver the necessary care. The initial response of the Soviet authorities was, "We don't need psychologists or psychiatrists; we need medication and surgical equipment." From their point of view, accepting mental health assistance was tantamount to admitting that they had "lost their minds." Or perhaps they suspected that Americans would come in and "read their thoughts" or "control their life." In fact, a Soviet official stated explicitly, "We lost some lives, arms and legs, but we did not lose our minds." This could be identified as resistance.

Resistance is a common phenomenon. The author has found that individuals will admit to their physical illnesses far more readily than to their emotional or psychological ones. In the case of Soviet administrators, it could also be identified as fear of the unknown, or more specifically, a fear of creating a situation in which they would have to express their innermost feelings to Americans, their "enemies." Lastly, they might fear assuming the dependent "sick role" by accepting help from Americans.

The resistance was much less profound in Southern Florida and in Southern California. Since this author had an established reputation and a demonstrated track record of research in a variety of outreach activities, a number of invitations were received from both disaster communities.

In Southern Florida, residents were able to get assistance through the Community Health Team, a mental health program funded by FEMA. They were the "Help on Wheels," going door-to-door in storm-ravaged areas, offering on-site counseling, referrals and practical advice. Some even handed out donated clothing from the back of their vans. The teams of four to seven professionals included nurses, mental health technicians, counselors and pediatric aides. They were recruited from the private sector and did not have to answer to a host of bureaucrats. They brought services to those who needed it, in leased vans, dispatched over cellular telephones. They responded to crises 24 hours-a-day.

The sum of $18.5 million was disbursed in crisis counseling grants to area mental health centers for treatment of disaster-related mental trauma. Other agencies, such as the Red Cross and other volunteer, religious and charitable organizations also fielded teams of professionals to provide help. The National Organization for Victim Assistance (NOVA) sent teams of professionals from Washington, D.C. to work with local providers during the day and hold community meetings, called debriefings, at night.

If resistance persists, it is essential to develop trust between professionals in the two countries or communities (one needing services and the other providing it). It is important to approach this matter from all possible angles and to express genuine concern and care in a non-threatening manner. In order to gain approval for entry into Soviet Armenia, this author approached the following institutions:

1. **Political:** Soviet and American Consulates, U.S. Congressmen, Mayors of Armenia.
2. **Religious:** Apostolic, Catholic and Protestant church leaders.
3. **Health/Psychiatry:** Ministries of Health and Education of Armenia and the Soviet Union; Chiefs of Psychiatry in Armenia and the Soviet Union; Presidents of Psychiatric Mental Health Organization in the United States, including the American Psychological and Psychiatric Associations, the International Society for Traumatic Stress Studies, the Orthopsychiatric Association, the William Alanson White Institute and many others.

After about six weeks of ongoing communication, negotiation and persistence, it became possible to travel to Soviet Armenia to continue the assessment phase and to develop and implement the Mental Health Outreach Program.

Preassessment Process

Prior to journeying to the disaster community, it is best to conduct all the necessary research pertaining to the type of natural disaster, the specific community needs and available community resources.

Prerequisites for an Outreach Program:

1. Consult with mental health experts in the field of disaster and trauma to gather Post-traumatic Stress Disorder (PTSD) assessment instruments and choose the most appropriate measure for the disaster at hand;
2. Initiate an intensive literature review on the impact of natural disaster (trauma) on the mental health of the survivor community;
3. Select an appropriate instrument for assessment; translate it into the native language of the impacted area and then translate it back to the source language to ensure accuracy of the translation;
4. Compile a roster of those mental health professionals fluent in the native language who are willing to devote their time;
5. Solicit financial assistance from institutions and foundations which could provide grants for this cause;
6. Collaborate with philanthropic organizations in the United States. In the case of Armenia, these included the Armenian General Benevolent Union, Armenian Missionary Association of America, Armenian Relief Society and Earthquake Relief Fund for Armenia;
7. Compile a list of and collaborate with other volunteer agencies providing assistance to the survivor communities, for example: Adventist Development and Relief Agency, American Red Cross, Ameri-Cares, CARE, Catholic Relief Services, Church World Services, Feed the Children, Lutheran World Relief, Mennonites Central Committee, National Medicare Care, People to People, Save the Children, Southern Baptist Foreign Mission Board, Werner Earhart Foundation, World Vision Relief and Development, Project Hope and many others;
8. Communicate and collaborate with mental health professionals in the disaster community.

Analysis of the Preassessment Phase

From the author's perspective, the emphasis had been placed consistently on the physical and material needs of the survivor community. Countries and organizations from around the world responded to the earthquake in Armenia with offers of aid ranging from orthopedic surgeons to equipment designed to detect signs of life under rubble. There was a feeling of excitement about extending a helping hand through what was once the Iron Curtain. There were also secondary gains from the earthquake for Armenia including intense publicity worldwide. Additionally, many Americans gave assistance out of feelings of over-compensation and in an attempt to undo past history by giving assistance to the enemy, in this instance, the Soviet Union. And it took this tragedy to bring the ten-month-old ethnic conflict between Armenia and Soviet Azerbaijan to the attention of the world community. All this goodwill and material assistance notwithstanding, it was apparent that no one was addressing the mental health and emotional needs of the survivor community, hence the development of the Mental Health Outreach Program.

In the case of Hurricane Andrew in Southern Florida, there were some attempts to help survivors cope with Post-traumatic stress symptomatology by establishing screening centers to evaluate those survivors who reached out for assistance. Southern California, on the other hand, was extremely well prepared to address the emotional and psychosocial needs of its survivor community. They already had well established, designated centers for counseling and psychiatric referrals.

Before the actual on site assessment it is advisable to review instruments measuring Post-traumatic Stress Disorder. The following PTSD assessment instruments were reviewed for their applicability for each disaster.

Assessment Instruments

The following Post-traumatic Stress Disorder assessment instruments were reviewed for their applicability:

1. The Structured Clinical Interview for DSM-III-R (SCID) (Spitzer et al., 1989)
2. Clinician Administered PTSD Scale (CAPS) (Blake et al., 1990)
3. The Diagnostic Interview Schedule (DIS) (Robbins et al., 1981)
4. The Impact of Event Scale (IES) (Horowitz et al., 1986)
5. The Brief Symptom Inventory (BSI) (Derogatis et al., 1983)
6. The Symptom Check List-90-R (Derogatis, 1977)
7. The Affect Balance Scale (ABS) (Bradburn, 1969)
8. The Reaction Index Scale (Frederick, 1986)

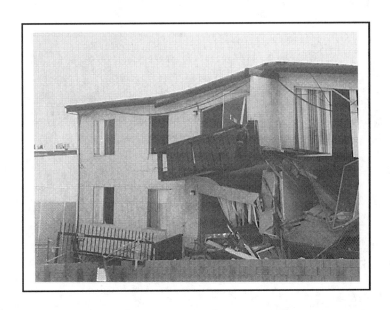

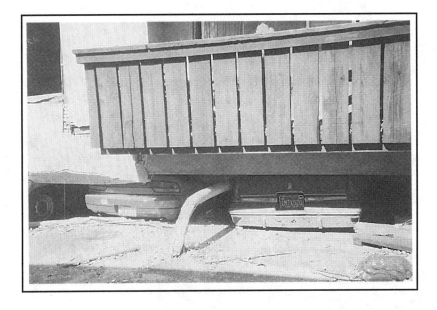

Two months hence: A residential dwelling demolished by the quake,
Northridge, California, March, 1994
Photographs by: Dr. Anie Sanentz Kalayjian

CHAPTER III

PHASE II

ON-SITE ASSESSMENT

CHAPTER III

Whatever authority I may have,
Rests solely in knowing how little I know.

Socrates

PHASE II

ASSESSMENT

The effectiveness of MHOP -- or any other outreach program -- is dependent on the rigor and thorough implementation of each phase. Assessment, the second phase in the MHOP, is the foundation of the outreach program, since this is where all the information about the actual impact of the disaster will be gathered first hand, on-site, unlike the pre-assessment phase, where the information is gathered through media, professional journals, newspapers, and secondary sources. A total assessment involves all areas of the surviving community: physical, psychological, sexual, economic, political, technological, cultural, and spiritual. Due to the chaotic situation in disaster environments, and time limitations, it is essential to focus on psychological assessment, especially since the cultural, physical, political, economic, and technological elements were reviewed in the pre-assessment phase.

Ideally, highly trained, expert mental health professionals should conduct the assessment. But in situations where those professionals are not available in sufficient numbers -- as was the case in Armenia -- one expert can train other professionals to collect some of the data (under supervision). Thus in Armenia, this author trained two psychiatrists to assist her in collecting the assessment data. This was not necessary in southern California or southern Florida, since highly trained and expert mental health professionals were available locally; also experts traveled from New York, Cincinnati, and other parts of the country.

The assessment phase begins immediately after the disaster, and it provides a foundation for analysis, community diagnosis, planning, and implementation. Depending on the severity of the disaster, community resources, and available personnel, assessment may range from one day to one month in duration. It is highly desirable to complete this phase as soon as possible, and as thoroughly as possible, so that one can move through the other phases in a timely fashion.

The assessment phase includes the following:

1. **Data Collection:** Collect data from a variety of sources: survivors, administrators, workers, government officials, etc.
2. **Data Validation:** Differentiate between factual and questionable data for accuracy. For example, in Leninakan, Armenia, some residents were convinced that what had happened had not been a quake, but was a cloaked nuclear attack perpetuated by the Soviet government in collaboration with the Azeri government. This data was not substantiated.
3. **Data Organization:** Cluster the data into groups of information that would help identify patterns of health or illness.
4. **Pattern Identification:** Check for patterns of information gathered and obtain additional data as needed to fill in the gaps in order to describe more clearly what the data means (Alfaro, 1985).

According to the Red Cross Manual on Disaster Health Services I, there are four stages of emotional response to natural disasters.

Stages of Emotional Response After Natural Disasters

1. **Denial:** During this first stage, survivors may deny the magnitude of the disaster; they may see and witness the incident, but may appear emotionally unaffected by it.
2. **Strong Emotional Response:** In this second stage, the survivor is emotionally aware of the problem and may feel overwhelmed and unable to cope with it. Common reactions during this stage are weeping, restlessness, sadness, anger, withdrawal and physical symptoms such as trembling, excessive sweating and speaking difficulties.
3. **Acceptance:** In this third stage, the survivor begins to accept the magnitude of the disaster and makes an appropriate effort to address it. Survivors feel more hopeful and goal-oriented. At this time, survivors may take more specific actions to help themselves and their families.
4. **Recovery:** Last but not least is the recovery stage, during which survivors feel that they have returned to their predisaster level of functioning. A sense of well-being and adjustment is restored and realistic memories of the traumatic experience are developed.

Need for On-Site Assessment

Although previous research studies, as well as consultation with mental health experts in this area, contributed to an understanding of the most common psychological responses to severe trauma, only through on-site assessment was the author able to comprehend the magnitude and severity of the Armenian quake. As one survivor stated, "If they had told me that there was a horror movie such as this (quake), I would not have believed it." In Armenia there were piles of steel, chunks of concrete, leveled buildings and the stench of corpses. People wearing inadequate clothing wandered about, eyes filled with tears of sadness, shock and disbelief. This was compounded by the terror of impending aftershocks, the decreasing hope of finding their loved ones, acute despair and asking "Why?" This was the same question asked by the survivors of Southern Florida, as well as Southern California, "Why?" and "Why us?"

The author found these disaster sites and interactions with the survivors both emotionally draining and professionally challenging. A prompt assessment of the survivor community was essential prior to diagnosis. Therefore, it was important to focus on target subgroups.

Based on this author's experience the most vulnerable groups impacted by disasters are the very young, adolescents, and the very old. Other groups exposed to tragedy because of their responsibilities in positions they hold are further affected by secondary trauma. Among those groups are: governmental bodies, administrators, clergy, media, and educators. In the caregiving professions, the most vulnerable are the health/mental health caregivers, and disaster relief workers.

Therefore, the following subgroups are recommended as the focus for the initial assessment after disasters.

1. Mental health professionals and health care providers in hospitals.
2. Educators and consultants in schools and community organizations.
3. Principals and administrative staff in schools and organizations.
4. Disaster relief workers at the disaster site.
5. Students in their schools, homes and hospitals.
6. Other survivors at home, work, on the streets, or in the markets and shops.
7. Government officials, Police and Armed Forces at their work sites.
8. Media personnel from radio, television and newspapers.
9. Personnel from religious and other voluntary service organizations.
10. Older adults in their residential and old age homes.

It is also essential to assess transportation and communication systems as to the level of disruption, as well as damages to hospitals (see Table 6), community centers, schools and churches.

Hospitals are an especially important part of the community's infrastructure before, during and after disasters. Not only do they serve the obvious, the ill, they also serve as valuable shelters with their multiple resources for food, life-enhancing equipment, and knowledgeable staff with a variety of backgrounds ranging from health and nutrition to legal and social services. Hospitals, as well as schools, should adhere strictly to building codes to ensure safety and minimal damage after disasters. For example, due to the destroyed hospitals in Leninakan, Armenia, the injured had to be transported to Yerevan, the capital, causing many more deaths, since the roads were adjured, and the traffic beyond description.

Hospitals Destroyed by Earthquakes in the Region of the Americas

HOSPITAL	COUNTRY	EARTHQUAKE
Kern Hospital	USA	Kern County, 1952
Hospital Traumatológico	Chile	Chile, 1960
Hospital de Valdivia	Chile	Chile, 1960
Elmendorf Hospital	USA	Alaska, 1964
Santa Cruz Hospital	USA	San Fernando, 1971
Olive View Hospital	USA	San Fernando, 1971
Veterans Administration Hospital	USA	San Fernando, 1971
Seguro Social	Nicaragua	Managua, 1972
Hospital Escalante Padilla	Costa Rica	San Isidro, 1983
Hospital Juárez	Mexico	Mexico, 1985
Centro Médico	Mexico	Mexico, 1985
Hospital Bloom	El Salvador	San Salvador, 1986
Hospital San Rafael	Cost Rica	Piedras Negras, 1990

Table 6

Mitigation of Disasters in Health Facilities
PAHO, (1993) Volume 4: Engineering Issues

Transportation:

- Air: airplanes, helicopters.
- Water: boats.
- Road: automobiles, buses, 4-wheel drive vehicles, horses, mules, or bridges.
- Railroad.

Communications:

- Telephone systems.
- Radio communications.
- Television.
- Human systems.
- Ham radios.

Community Facilities:

- Hospitals.
- Houses of worship.
- Schools.
- Community centers.
- Municipal buildings.

Common Sources of Information:

- Civil defense.
- United Nations representative agencies.
- Red Cross.
- Armed forces.
- Heads of regional organizations.
- Heads of other voluntary organizations.
- Government agencies.

Assessment Instruments

Diane Kupelian, Ph.D.

As clinical experience, knowledge and theoretical models concerning Post-traumatic stress syndromes have grown, instruments for measuring and describing the construct have become more available and more sophisticated. Many of the existing measures of Post-traumatic symptomatology are oriented towards combat veterans, reflecting a major impetus to development in this field. However, some measures are more general in scope and equally applicable for assessing those who were exposed to a traumatic stress from natural disaster. What follows is a short description of some selected assessment instruments that may prove useful for either clinical research or therapeutic purposes.

Interview Assessments

The Structured Clinical Interview for DSM-III-R (SCID) (Spitzer, et al. 1989) comes in an interview series, with a separate SCID-PTSD module. [Note: An updated version of the SCID-PTSD module keyed to DSM-IV criteria is available through the American Psychiatric Association, but because the most extensive reliability information is available for the version keyed to the DSM-III-R, that version is discussed here]. Each module of the series is keyed directly to the DSM-III-R criteria and is designed to be administered by a trained mental health clinician. The interviewing clinician assesses the presence, absence or sub-threshold presence of each symptom. This can be assessed currently and for past occurrences of disorder. The SCID I and SCID-II cover Axis I (clinical syndromes) and Axis II (personality disorders). The entire series is available in versions designed for inpatients, outpatients and people not identified as patients (non-patient version). The fact that diagnosis in each module is accomplished by a clinician to Diagnostic Statistical Manual (DSM) criteria gives this measure criterion validity at least to the DSM definition of the given disorder.

The PTSD module of the SCID may be the most commonly used clinical interview for assessing Post-traumatic stress syndromes. Because it is frequently used, research studies employing the SCID-PTSD module are more easily comparable, and there is also a growing body of information on the psychometric properties of the test. Some reliability data for the PTSD module of the SCID are available from the National Vietnam Veterans Readjustment Study (NVVRS) (reported in Weiss, 1993). Audio tapes and notes of 440 interviews with veterans

59

using the SCID-PTSD module were reviewed by one of the five expert clinicians in the NVVRS. For diagnoses of current PTSD, there were only 11 rediagnoses or .025 percent. But for diagnoses of lifetime PTSD, there were only 8 rediagnoses or .018 percent. Interrater reliability was investigated for 30 cases randomly selected from the original 440. The statistic used was the Kappa coefficient for the measurement of observer agreement for qualitative, categorical data (Cohen, 1960). The level of interrater reliability was excellent, with Kappa coefficients for lifetime PTSD computed to be .94, and for the current diagnosis to be .87.

In another study, the SCID-PTSD module was used with a geriatric population of Armenian genocide survivors (Kupelian, 1993). In that study, 22 of 68 interviews were randomly selected for a measure of inter-rater reliability, which again, was in the NVVRS study above, was generally excellent. The Cohen's Kappa coefficients for the lifetime PTSD diagnosis in this case were also computed separately for the three major symptom clusters. Kappa coefficients were computed for lifetime intrusion symptoms to be .85, for lifetime avoidance symptoms were .88, and the lifetime arousal symptoms to be an acceptable .60. The Kappa for current intrusion symptoms was computed to be excellent .92 (very good for current avoidance symptoms, .76, and acceptable for current arousal symptoms, .60).

The SCID-PTSD module appears to be a reliable instrument (according to Kalayjian, 1994) with criterion validity to the DSM definition of the disorder. As more studies offering reliability information broken down by the three major symptoms groups of PTSD become available, the relative stability of those item groups will be better described. The SCID-PTSD module is efficiently focused on the current delineation of the disorder. Other measures might also be used to investigate co-morbidity and aspects accompanying the disorder not currently included in the definition. If time and availability of trained mental health professionals permits, administration of other parts of the SCID could provide a thorough investigation.

A somewhat more extensive structured interview is the *Clinician Administered PTSD Scale (CAPS)* (Blake, Weathers, Hagy, Kaloupek, Klauminzer, Charney, & Keane, 1990). Like the SCID-PTSD module, it is also keyed directly to the 17 symptoms of the DSM-III-R criteria. However, the CAPS also includes eight associated symptoms the authors derived from the PTSD literature and five global rating scales for various dimensions of functioning and assessment.

The assessment for each criterion on the CAPS is not limited to a judgement of the presence or absence of the symptom. Rather, the assessment for each item is accomplished on two scales: frequency of the symptom and the most extreme intensity of that symptom. The combination of frequency and intensity for 25 PTSD-related symptoms allows for patternings of the symptom picture, with a sensitivity to the degree of distress. Repeated administrations could track the course of the disorder in some detail, a feature which could be useful in research as well as in assessing treatment. The increased scope and detail of the CAPS, however, may require a longer administration time. The scale was constructed with behavioral anchors for each item of the scale, with the idea that specially trained nonprofessionals could administer the CAPS. This practical factor may balance the increased time required to administer the interview.

In a study of 123 veterans, the authors of the CAPS report test-retest reliability ranging from .90 to .98 for the 17 DSM-III-R criteria and ranging from .77 to .96 for the three symptom cluster of intrusion, avoidance and arousal (reported in Blake, et al. in press). Blake, et al. also report excellent overall internal consistency for the major 17 symptoms (alpha=.94), and a strong correlation with other measures of PTSD. The CAPS appears to measure the diagnostic construct with consistency and reliability to the criteria set by DSM-III-R. In addition, it measures some wider symptom areas associated with the disorder but not included in the formal definition of PTSD.

The Diagnostic Interview Schedule (DIS) (Robins, et al. 1981) was originally devised as an epidemiological instrument to be administered by non-professionals in a community setting. The Disaster Supplement (DS) for assessing Post-traumatic syndromes was added later (Robbins & Smith, 1983). Although the DIS/DS is available in several languages and well used, there is little published validity data on that version. The NVVRS used a version of the DIS module to assess PTSD, and found that as the subject population changed, the calculated validity of the instrument also changed (reported in Blake, et al. in press and Weiss, 1993). The scale appeared valid in a small group of treatment-seeking veterans (sensitivity = .87; specificity = .73; concurrent validity with the SCID-PTSD module, kappa = .64). However, with the larger group of 440 veterans in the community, the validity declined markedly (sensitivity = .22; specificity = .98; concurrent validity kappa = .26). It may be that this measure is effective with people seeking help, and may yet prove useful as a screening instrument. If this is used cautiously and along with other measures for those seeking help in the wake of a disaster it could prove effective.

Self-Report Measures

The Impact of Event Scale (IES) (Horowitz, et al. 1979) is one of the most frequently used measures of the cognitive symptoms of Post-traumatic stress. It is a 15-item self-report measure that summarizes the impact of a specific trauma on the two major cognitive dimensions of intrusion and avoidance. The scale is not keyed directly to the descriptive DSM criteria; rather, it grew out of the theory that Post-traumatic symptomatology is based on the phasic interplay of cognitive intrusion and avoidance, which continues until the individual assimilates the traumatic experience. This instrument has repeatedly demonstrated good validity and reliability in psychometric studies across survivor groups. For example, bereaved adults (Zilberg, et al. 1982), Isreali combat soldiers (Schwarzwald, et al. 1987), and survivors of disasters at sea (Joseph, et al. 1992; Joseph, et al. 1993).

Because theoretical underpinnings of the IES postulate that the measured symptoms should change over time, it was constructed to be a continuous measure so that it could be sensitive to assess change. It is easily administered and scored and is a well respected instrument for post-disaster research or therapeutic work.

The Brief Symptom Inventory (BSI) (Derogatis & Melisaratos, 1983) is a 53 item self-report symptom inventory that taps nine primary symptom dimension subscales: somatization, obsessive-compulsive symptoms, interpersonal sensitivity, depression, anxiety, hostility, phobic anxiety, paranoid ideation and psychoticism. This measure also renders three global indices of distress. Test-retest reliability ranges from .68 to .91 on the various scales (Derogatis, 1992), and Cronbach's alpha ranged between .71 and .85 (Derogatis & Melisaratos, 1983). Construct validity in the acceptable to good range was found in a factor analytic study (Derogatis, 1992). Two screening studies have found that an initial administration of the BSI correctly identified medical patients experiencing psychological difficulties (Kuhn, Bell, Seligson, Laufer, & Linder 1988; Zabora, Smith-Wilson, Fetting, & Engerlin,. 1990). This is a general screening instrument which is easily administered, scored and very practical for quick assessments.

The Symptom Check List-90-R (SCL-90-R) (Derogatis, 1977) is the original, longer version from which the BSI was derived and affords the same array of information. It has demonstrated acceptable validity and reliability (Derogatis & Cleary, 1977a; Derogatis & Cleary, 1977b). There is a recent exploratory use of a sub-scale which may be of particular interest in the context of PTSD assessment. Two studies have isolated a subset SCL-90-R item which has shown promise in identifying women suffering from crime related Post-traumatic stress disorder (CR-PTSD) (Saunders, et al. 1990; Arata, et al. 1991). The fact that individuals do not apparently need to make a connection between a particular trauma and their current experience of symptoms can be valuable in a screening situation where this might be an additional concern.

Another very easily administered and frequently used self-report measure is the *Affect Balance Scale (ABS)* (Bradburn, 1969. It is simply a list of adjectives that are endorsed on a five point Likert-type scale and does not require a reference to the traumatic situation to assess mood state. It renders scores for positive affect, negative affect and affect balance and is built on a theory of assessing well-being.   Recent studies have generally indicated acceptable reliability and validity (Kempen, 1992; Liang, 1985).   Although it does not measure trauma related symptoms, the ease of administration for this mood measurement makes this a good choice for inclusion along with other assessments.

The above is a short summary of selected available measures for research (except *The Reaction Index Scale*, Frederick, 1986, which is discussed next) for clinical work with victims of traumatic stress. It is probably best to use a combination of measures whenever possible, matching their attributes and requirements to the demands of the situation as it presents itself. Some will be more useful as a quick screen in the urgency immediately following a disaster, some as an in-depth assessment at follow-up and some might best be used in both situations as a measure of change.

A Discussion of the Assessment Instruments Utilized

Adults: The clarity and brevity of the *Reaction Index Scale* made it the instrument of choice for this author, given a chaotic disaster milieu in which expeditious assessment was requisite for the effective implementation of MHOP. This 28 item instrument for adults (20 items for children) had a scoring range of zero to four for each item, with a total of eighty possible points. Scoring was bi-directional. Both parts of the instruments (adult and child) were translated into Eastern Armenian, the language of the survivor community. Based on the effectiveness of this instrument, the author utilized it in the subsequent disasters in Southern Florida as well as in Southern California.

Children: Structured and unstructured drawings were utilized to assess the level of trauma in children under the age of ten. A structured drawing is one in which the child is given specific directions as to what to draw. In this situation, the children were first instructed to draw their houses at the time of the quake and to include themselves, members of their families and anything else they considered significant. Then, they were asked to draw their future homes. For unstructured drawings, in contrast, children are given little or no instruction as to what to draw. The latter form was used when children were hesitant or resistant to draw under the structured method. After the 1972 Buffalo Creek Dam disaster in West Virginia, children's drawings were used as therapeutic modes of intervention (Newman, 1976). On February 26, 1972, heavy rains caused a dam in Logan County, West Virginia to collapse, flooding the numerous coal mining homesites dotting the narrow Buffalo Creek Valley below. The disaster killed 125 people and left thousands without shelter.

The Reaction Index Scale was also used with adolescents in Armenia, Southern Florida and Southern California as a diagnostic tool.

Play as an Assessment Instrument: Play therapy was used as a diagnostic tool with those young children who refused to draw and/or could not verbally communicate their fears and experiences about the quake. Houses, trees, animals, cars and significant figures were utilized to set the scene of the event. This procedure had been advocated as an intervention technique by mental health clinicians after the Nicaraguan earthquake in 1972 (Cohen & Ahearn, 1980). Puppets were also used as a means to present significant others during the play, and where puppets were not available, children fashioned puppets from pillows, sheets and crayons.

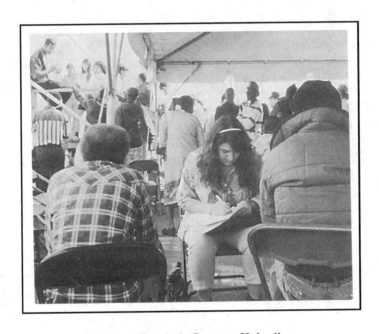

Three months hence: Dr. Anie Sanentz Kalayjian
      Conducting an assessment in
      Homestead, Florida
      December, 1992

CHAPTER IV

PHASE III
ANALYSIS

CHAPTER IV

Facts, after all, are like the moon: they derive their light and hence their import from an external force.

Kasper D. Naegle

PHASE III

ANALYSIS

The analysis phase follows preassessment and assessment sequentially. Data from preassessment and assessment phases are gathered, clustered and organized for the analysis. Analysis is a cognitive process, using critical thinking and the information gathered from the two previous phases to reach accurate and definitive diagnoses, or to give impressions of the surviving community.

Data from the preassessment phase are used as a theoretical basis for clustering and organizing data regarding the surviving community and the overall environment. Data from the assessment phase are examined to identify the specific client or community strengths and deficits, available and desirable resourses and the overall readiness and motivation.

The analysis phase will lead professionals into the diagnosis phase, which then will guide them into planning, implementation, evaluation and remodification.

The Diagnostic and Statistical Manual of the American Psychiatric Association (DSM-IV, 1994), is a manual used to categorize, organize and label professionals' clinical impressions. Based on the DSM-IV, disasters and mass trauma may cause PTSD, which is categorized as an anxiety disorder defined below.

Definition of PTSD

According to the DSM-IV (1994), Post-traumatic Stress Disorder (PTSD) (309.81) is categorized amongst anxiety disorders and it has the following six categories:

A.   The person has been exposed to a traumatic event in which both of the following were present:

1. The person has experienced, witnessed or was confronted with an event or events that involved actual or threatened death or serious injury or a threat to the physical integrity of self or others.
2. The person's response involved intense fear, helplessness or horror. Note: In children, it may be expressed instead by disorganized or agitated behavior.

B.   The traumatic event is persistently re-experienced in one or more of the following ways:

1. Recurrent, intrusive, and distressing recollections of the event, including images, thoughts or perceptions. Note: In young children, repetitive play may occur in which themes or aspects of the trauma are expressed.
2. Recurrent, distressing dreams of the event. Note: In children, there may be frightening dreams without recognizable content.
3. Acting or feeling as if the traumatic event were recurring, which may involve a sense of reliving the experience, illusions, hallucinations and dissociative flashback episodes (including those that occur on awakening or when intoxicated). Note: In young children, trauma specific reenactment may occur.
4. Intense psychological distress at exposure to internal or external cues that symbolize or resemble an aspect of the traumatic event.
5. Physiologic reactivity on exposure to internal or external cues that symbolize or resemble an aspect of the traumatic event.

C.   Persistent avoidance of stimuli associated with the trauma and numbing of general responsiveness (not present before the trauma), as indicated by three or more of the following:

1. Efforts to avoid thoughts, feelings or conversations associated with the trauma.
2. Efforts to avoid activities, places or people that arouse recollections of the trauma.
3. Inability to recall an important aspect of the trauma.
4. Markedly diminished interest or participation in significant activities.
5. Feeling of detachment or estrangement from others.
6. Restricted range of affect (e.g., unable to have loving feelings).
7. Sense of a foreshortened future (e.g., does not expect to have a career, marriage, children or a normal life span).

D.   Persistent symptoms of increased arousal (not present before that trauma), as indicated by at least two of the following:

1. Difficulty falling or staying asleep.
2. Irritability or outbursts of anger.
3. Difficulty concentrating.
4. Hypervigilance.
5. Exaggerated startled response.

E.   Duration of the disturbance (symptoms in B, C and D) is more than one
      month.

F.   The disturbance causes clinically significant distress or impairment in
      social, occupational or other important areas of functioning.
      (**Note:** Reprinted with permission from the American Psychiatric Association)

Acute PTSD is specified as the duration of symptoms for less than three months, as opposed to chronic PTSD with a duration of symptoms three months or more.

According to DSM-IV (1994), in PTSD the stressor must be of an extreme (e.g. life-threatening) nature. In contrast, in Adjustment Disorder, the stressor is not an extreme nature, and is not necessarily life-threatening (e.g. spouse leaving, being fired).

Not all psychopathology resulting from an exposure to an extreme stressor is necessarily PTSD. Symptoms of avoidance, numbing and increased arousal that existed before the exposure to the stressor do not meet criteria for PTSD diagnosis. These symptoms may be other diagnoses such as a Mood Disorder or another Anxiety Disorder. It could even be that the symptoms exhibited in response to an extreme stressor meet other diagnoses (e.g. Brief Psychotic Disorder, Major Depressive Disorder, etc.). These diagnoses should be assigned instead of the PTSD. For the purposes of this manual, the author has focused on the PTSD as the clinical diagnosis.

Highly trained and expert mental health professionals should conduct the analysis. Especially since the PTSD scale as well as other assessment instruments are utilized to conduct the analysis phase. But, in situations where those professionals are not available in sufficient numbers - as was found earlier in the assessment phase - one expert can train other professionals to complete the analysis phase.

The analysis phase begins immediately after the assessment phase is completed and must continue until satisfactory, accurate and definitive diagnoses have been reached. Analysis may resume as new and additional information is gathered.

Armenia

Analysis

Psychological and behavioral symptoms were first assessed systematically six to eight weeks after the earthquake due to difficulties obtaining access visas. Over two hundred adults and two hundred adolescents and children constituted the assessment sample. The site of the assessments varied. Several different layers of the community were observed in their natural environments, i.e., school age children and adolescents in their classrooms during recess, in hospitals, shelters or in their homes; adults at their work places (if they were still employed), in hospitals, at government shelters or at the homes of their relatives. Geographically, emphasis was placed on the quake zone in Armenia: Leninakan, Kirovakan, Spitak and a few of the villages that were en route to the larger cities. In Southern Florida emphasis was placed on Homestead, Coconut Grove, Cutler Ridge, South Miami and other areas in Dade, Broward and Collier Counties. In California emphasis was placed on Northridge, Van Nuys, Hollywood and Glendale. Data from the assessment was used for this analysis.

Short-Term Effects of Disaster Manifested in Children and Adolescents in Armenia

The Most Common Psychological Symptoms Manifested by Children After a Natural Disaster:

1. Separation anxiety: excessive clinging to parents, or significant others, intensifying at night.
2. Refusing to sleep or be left alone.
3. Refusing to go to school.
4. Conduct disorder.
5. Regressive behavior: thumb-sucking, enuresis or clinging behaviors.
6. Hyperactivity.
7. Withdrawal.
8. Inability to concentrate.
9. Somatic complaints: stomach ache, headache, joint aches, etc.
10. Sleep disturbances: bad dreams, frequent awakenings or difficulty falling asleep.

Assessment of Children:

The most common psychological and behavioral symptoms detected in children up to seven years of age are mentioned above. Eighty-six percent of the children interviewed or observed (N=122, F=60%), displayed at least four of the following ten symptoms: separation anxiety intensified during the night; refusing to go to school; refusing to sleep or to be left alone; conduct disorders; sleep disturbances manifested by bad dreams, frequent awakenings, difficulty falling asleep; regressive behavior manifested by thumb sucking, enuresis and clinging behaviors; hyperactivity; withdrawal; inability to concentrate; and somatic complaints. Utilizing the Reaction Index Scale (Frederick, 1986), 82.8% of the adolescents interviewed (N=62, F=55%) scored over fifty, indicating severe levels of Post-traumatic Stress Disorder (PTSD). The most common psychological and behavioral symptoms observed in adolescents were as follows: withdrawal, lack of concentration, aggressive tendencies, nightmares, unusually poor grades in courses in which they had excelled prior to the earthquake, irritability and increased reports of episodic daydreaming.

Assessment of Adolescents

The Most Common Psychological Symptoms Manifested by Adolescents After Natural Disasters

1. Withdrawal.
2. Anger.
3. Increased aggression.
4. Regression.
5. Sleep disturbances.

6. Nightmares.
7. Increased daydreaming.
8. Inability to concentrate.
9. Irritability.
10. Poor grades in courses excelled in prior to the disaster.

Responses of adolescents differ somewhat from those exhibited by children and adults. Although a few research findings indicate the short-lived nature of responses by adolescents to disaster, very few studies focus on the frequency and the intensity of those responses. Milgram and colleagues (1988) studied seventh graders nine months after a school bus disaster and found they had very few psychological symptoms. Nader et al. (1990) assessed children and adolescents after a sniper attack at their school and similarly found their Post-traumatic stress symptoms decreased within 14 months after the trauma.

70

Adolescent disaster stress response differs from those of adults and children. Developmentally, adolescents are in a unique and inherently stressful stage, with distinct emotional and psychological needs (Garrison et al., 1987; Rutter et al., 1986). In addition, adolescents do not have the advantage of increased age and multiple life experiences to rely on, as do adults. In the one-to-one interviews with the adult survivors of Hurricane Andrew, there was a repeated theme of benefiting from previous experiences. Gleser et al. (1981) studied white children and adolescents one-year-and-a-half to two years after the Buffalo Creek disaster and found that disaster stress increased from childhood to adolescence. They also found that 20% adolescents (N=82) 12 to 15 years of age reported anxiety; 30% reported depression. Prior healthy coping experiences, a viable family support system and low level of life event stress are considered to be prerequisites to a healthy adolescent response to a disaster (Andrews et al., 1978). According to Andrews et al., those meeting the above-mentioned prerequisites had a 13% risk for psychiatric difficulties, while those not meeting the prerequisites exhibited a 43% rate of psychiatric complications.

According to Hardin et al. (1994), who studied 1482 South Carolina high school students a year after Hurricane Hugo, as exposure to the hurricane increased, so did symptoms of psychological distress. However, the study by Hardin et al. (1994) was limited, as are almost all the studies on natural disasters, by its inability to compare the baseline psychological distress scores of adolescents before and after the disaster. As a whole, the study revealed that social support and self-efficacy are inversely related to psychological distress, which reinforced studies of Baum et al. (1983), Fleming et al. (1982) and Murphy (1987). Social support was even a better protector against psychological distress than self-efficacy, reinforcing studies by Fleming et al. (1982), Berndt and Ladd (1989), and others, who found peer support to be essential for teens in distress.

Assessment of Adults

The Most Common Psychological Symptoms Manifested by Adults After Natural Disasters:

1. Uncertainty and fear.
2. Anger.
3. Feeling tense, edgy and jumpy.
4. Loss of appetite.
5. Sleep disturbances and nightmares.
6. Loss of interest or inability to engage in sexual activities.
7. Withdrawal.
8. Loss of concentration.
9. Inability to make decisions.
10. Aggression turned inward and outward.

Two hundred twelve adults (62% female) were interviewed or assessed in Armenia. The Reaction Index Scale was utilized. Over eighty percent (80%) scored in excess of 50 on the Reaction Index Scale, indicating severe levels of Post-traumatic Stress Disorder (PTSD). Over eighty percent (80%) of those interviewed admitted to having at least five of the psychological symptoms listed.

Meaning in Trauma

According to another research study conducted by this author six weeks after the earthquake in Armenia where survivors were asked an open-ended question eliciting the meaning they had attributed to the earthquake, twenty percent (20%) attributed a positive value and meaning to the disaster (Kalayjian, 1991c). This is congruent with Quarantelli's (1985) notion that disaster survivors are primarily attempting to cope with the meaning of the trauma and with Frankl's (1978) assertion that meaning is available under any condition, even the worst conceivable one. This is somewhat contrary to Figley's (1985) belief that one of the fundamental questions a victim needs to answer in order to become a survivor is "Why did it happen?" This author's research findings indicated that a question of that type forced the survivor to remain in the past, in the role of a victim, without a rational or satisfactory answer. It also left the survivor filled with feelings of self-induced guilt and therefore, trapped in a cycle of destructive behavior. Viktor Frankl, the author of *Man's Search for Meaning*, in a personal communication, labeled this type of "why" question as the "wrong question." Any question that begins with a "why" has a built-in presumption that there is someone responsible for the incident. In this case, it was the natural disaster. Those survivors from Armenia, Florida, and California were preoccupied with the question of "Why did this happen?" were dissatisfied with the scientific answer that "the plates moved, pressure was built up and finally the tension was released." Survivors, especially in California and Florida, were informed regarding the "why's" of the earthquake and the hurricane, but some of the them chose to remain in the "why" mode of thinking. Interestingly, these were the survivors who remained helpless, more depressed and showed higher scores on the PTSD Reaction Index Scale.

In Armenia:

In Armenia, those survivors who were preoccupied with the "why's" were uninterested in the scientific explanation. They countered with the questions, "Why us? What have we done to deserve this?" This question "Why was my child, my parents or my school affected?" implied that trauma and disaster happen to bad, sinful or unworthy people, attributing a negative meaning to the disaster.

Survivors who attributed a positive meaning focused instead on the present moment and the meaningful experiences they had gained by helping or receiving help from one another and from the world. As one survivor from Armenia stated, "Look at how the world has come to help us (the Armenians), the closed Soviet system has opened its doors, there is more communication, caring and sharing."

According to this author's research findings (1991c), twenty percent (20%) of the survivors in Armenia were convinced that they were indomitable, echoing the words of Nietzsche (1956), who said, "That which does not kill me makes me stronger."

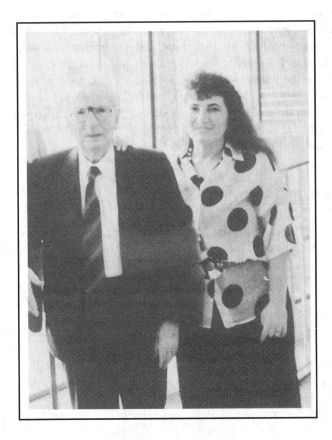

Dr. Anie Sanentz Kalayjian
with
Dr. Viktor Frankl
(Author of *Man's Search for Meaning*)
At the Eighth World Congress of Logotherapy, San Jose, California
July, 1989
Reprinted with permission from the *Armenian Reporter*.

Analysis In California:

In Southern California close to forty percent (40%) of the survivors uttered statements indicating the establishment of positive meaning in their experiences of the earthquake. Typical statements ranged from "I went through many quakes in my life, I always replace all the china and the broken crystal. This time is different, this time I learned something about life's meaning. This time I'm not going to replace the unnecessary crystal. I now value my friends and family, and will put all my energy to be with them," and "Materials are here today and gone tomorrow, from now on I am going to invest in people," "This (quake) was a good lesson to me of life, not material. I did not lose my life and the lives of the loved ones, thank God, and that is what counts."

Analysis In Southern Florida:

In Southern Florida, over thirty percent (30%) of the survivors interviewed by this author indicated that they had established positive meaning in their experiences of the hurricane. Responses such as "Although I felt vulnerable to Mother Nature, talking and working with friends and fellow employees I found the most meaningful and "Helping friends and neighbors are most important in life" were indicative of the meanings attributed to their traumatic experiences.

Respondents who found meaning in their trauma measured much lower on the Reaction Index Scale, indicating lower levels of Post-traumatic Stress Disorder. They also reached acceptance which is an essential step in the move toward resolving an existential crisis. The acceptance stage, as defined by Kubler-Ross (1969), is neither happy nor sad. It is devoid of feeling, a passive acquiescence to the tragic triad of human existence: pain, guilt and death (Frankl, 1962).

Long-Term Effects of Natural Disasters

According to van der Kolk (1987), until the last decade the notion that massive stress may, in some circumstances, leave a psychogenic syndrome in its wake was not widely accepted. Although both natural and man-made disasters have been with us for centuries, only in the last decade has a formal diagnosis for Post-traumatic Stress Disorder been agreed upon and added to the *Diagnostic Statistical Manual*.

Although there is a plethora of literature addressing long-term psychosocial effects of man-made disaster, e.g., wars, very few research studies address the same impact of natural disasters. Prior to the development of the term Post-traumatic Stress Disorder, other terms were utilized describing the continuing nervous problems of soldiers returning from wars: shell shock, combat fatigue and organic brain damage. The author found no comparable terms used describing the psychosocial symptoms of survivors of natural disasters.

One natural disaster whose survivors were studied systematically is the Buffalo Creek, West Virginia, dam collapse of 1972. Gleser et al. (1981) followed some survivors for up to five years post-disaster. Green et al. (1990) studied those survivors two, five and then 14 years after the disaster. The latter study's goal was to determine whether there were lingering psychological effects of the dam collapse in the second decade, focusing on longitudinal stability and change.

Studies of the Buffalo Creek dam collapse and the Beverly Hills Supper Club fire conducted by Gleser et al. (1981), Green et al. (1983) showed decreases in several types of pathology between two and five years after the flood and between one and two years after the fire. According to Green et al. (1990) in the case of the Beverly Hills fire, however, those survivors who witnessed the fire showed a significant increase in hostility, as measured by the SCL-90 one to two years after the fire, suggesting a latency period or delayed onset of some symptoms. According to Green et al. (1990), there was a highly significant decrease in symptoms over the 12 year period.

According to this author's one year follow-up research in Armenia, earthquake survivors exhibited a significant increase in anger and helplessness, as well as an increased consumption of alcohol and reports of violence in the family (Kalayjian, 1994a). This may have been partially due to the ongoing trauma with Azerbaijan over the enclave of Nagorno-Karabagh, the struggle for democracy and independence and the economic hardship caused by the Azeri blockade.

Tierney and Baisden (1979), who studied the psychological effects of the 1974 tornado in Xenia, Ohio, found a decreased alcohol consumption level and improved relationships with friends and family 18 months following the tornado. They also noted reports of physical illness and depression.

Phifer et al. (1988), who studied elderly survivors of natural disasters, described a seasonal trend in symptoms following a flood in Southeastern Kentucky. The symptoms peaked in the first spring after the incident, decreased in the fall and increased to a lesser degree the following spring. This seasonal trend was evident in those survivors who had high personal losses and high community destruction.

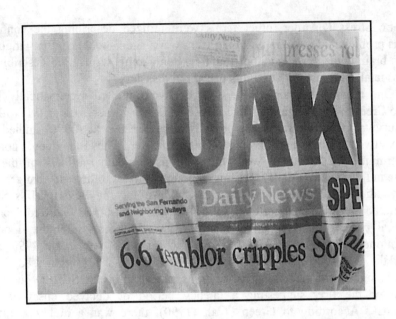

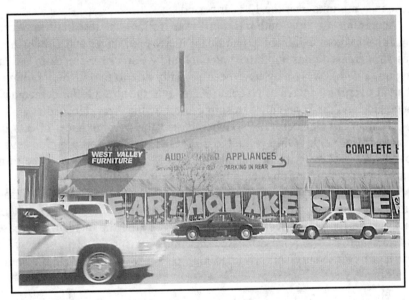

Less than two months hence: Valley entrepreneurs
making the best of a bad situation.
Northridge, California
March 1, 1994.

Photographs by: Dr. Anie Sanentz Kalayjian

CHAPTER V

PHASE IV

COMMUNITY DIAGNOSES

CHAPTER V

A good part of the struggles of mankind center around the single task of finding an expedient accommodation-one, that is, that will bring happiness-between this claim of the individual and the cultural claim of the group; and one of the problems that touches the fate of humanity is whether such an accommodation can be reached by means of some particular form of civilization or whether the conflict is irreconcilable.

Sigmund Freud
Civilization and Its Discontents

PHASE IV

COMMUNITY DIAGNOSES

Community diagnosis is a statement describing the community's response to the disaster. Diagnoses are utilized as classifications to express conclusions based on the data gathered in the preassessment, assessment and the analysis phases.

Diagnoses generally are abstract and broad labels, or definitions of phenomena that health professionals use to help clients, as well as communities, to change and improve. These labels, or inferences, are utilized to assist professionals in their planning and implementations of care.

A thorough analysis of the assessment of the impact of the earthquake in Armenia and individual interview conducted by this author revealed several diagnoses.

Diagnoses in Armenia Post 1988 Earthquake:

1. 86% of the children interviewed had severe PTSD.
2. 83% of the adolescents interviewed had severe PTSD.
3. 81% of the adults interviewed had severe PTSD.
4. 80% of the teachers interviewed in Leninakan were survivors themselves.
5. Over 79% of the leaders and government officials interviewed from the quake zone were survivors themselves.
6. 80% of the mental health professionals interviewed from the quake zone exhibited signs of burnout.

78

7. 98% of the survivors in the earthquake zone did not have a mental health professional available to provide care.
8. There was only one community mental health outpatient clinic in Leninakan.
9. Spitak and some 56 affected villages had no mental health providers or centers.
10. There were 39.2 physicians for every 10,000 people in Armenia (Ministry of Health, Moscow, 1991).

PSYCHOLOGICAL IMPACT

of

HURRICANE ANDREW

IMMEDIATE	3 MONTHS	6 MONTHS
* Shock	* Hopelessness	* Uncertainty
* Helping One Another	* Helplessness	* Frustration
* Fear	* Anger	* Abusive Relationships
	* Fear	* Increased Fear
		* Despair
		* Apathy

(Kalayjian, 1993)

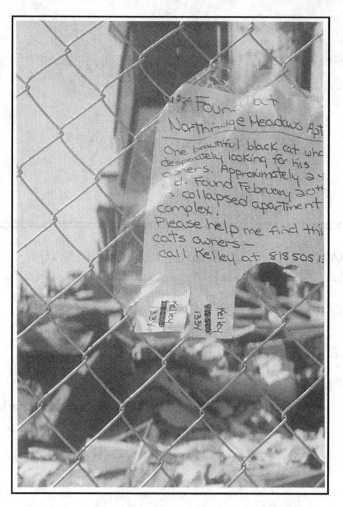

Two months hence: A homemade flyer taped on a wire fence
                   reads: "Found in a Northridge Meadows
                   apartment: One beautiful black cat who is
                   desperately looking for his owners.
                   Approximately 24 mo. old. Found
                   February 20th in collapsed apartment
                   complex. Please help me find this cat's
                   owners - - call Kelly at # ....."
                   Northridge, California
                   March 1, 1994

Kelly's effort illustrates how calamities bring out the best in us all.
        Photograph by: Dr. Anie Sanentz Kalayjian

Community Diagnoses in Southern Florida Post Hurricane Andrew:

1. 89% of the children interviewed had severe PTSD.
2. 86% of the adolescents interviewed had severe PTSD.
3. 86% of the adults interviewed had severe PTSD.
4. 80% of the disaster workers interviewed had severe PTSD.
5. Over 70% of the health care workers had severe PTSD.
6. Over 50% of the teachers and educators interviewed had severe PTSD.
7. Over 50% of the contractors were from outside of Florida and further aggravated the trauma to the community by misusing trust.
8. Many residents decided to leave the community, thereby increasing the stress of rebuilding for the few families remaining behind.
9. The majority of the survivors expressed frustration due to not receiving emergency aid promptly.
10. The closing of Homestead Air Force Base caused many to relocate.

Community Diagnoses in Southern California Post 1994 Earthquake:

1. The quake was experienced as the 'Big One.'
2. Community was organized in their efforts for relief and aid disbursement.
3. 34% of those interviewed expressed plans for relocation.
4. 67% of the adults interviewed had severe PTSD.
5. 88% of the children interviewed had severe PTSD.
6. 50% of the mental health workers had signs of PTSD.
7. 30% of the teachers and educators in the affected area had severe PTSD.
8. No outside contractors were present.
9. Survivors were content with the relief efforts.
10. 98% of the residents interviewed complained about the additional traffic jam due to the quake.

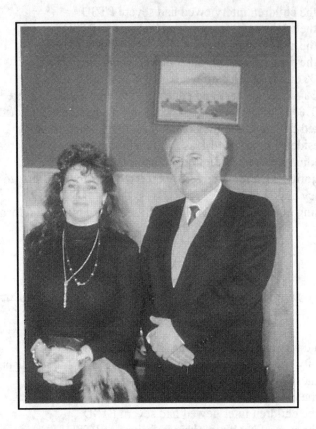

One month hence: Meeting with Mr. Garen Dallakian, President
of the Committee for Cultural Relations with
Armenians Abroad, Dr. Kalayjian secures the
official support of the then Soviet Armenian
Government.
Yerevan, Armenia
January, 1989

Reprinted with permission from the *Armenian Reporter*

83

CHAPTER VI

PHASE V

PLANNING

CHAPTER VI

When schemes are laid in advance,
it is surprising how often circumstances fit in with them.

Sir William Osler

PHASE V

PLANNING

In planning, the fifth phase of the MHOP, the professional determines from the first four phases what needs to be done, in what order, how it will be done, and who will be responsible for the delivery. Information from the preassessment, assessment, analysis and diagnosis, are utilized in the planning phase. It is this phase in which the ordering of information and its use is decided.

Planning is the prioritizing needs and organizing resources of individuals and their community. Planning provides the process of implementation. Planning is comprised of two components short-term and long-term.

Short-terms goals are developed to address the acute needs of the community. This begins immediately after the analysis and continues until the goals have been met. Long-term plans address rehabilitation, education and training needs of the community. This plan begins after the completion of the short-term goals and continues as long as necessary. The specific time frames differ for each of these goals based on the type of disaster, predisaster mental health status, needs of the community, desired end result and resources available to the community.

1. Short-term planning

In this phase the goal is to elevate the immediate psychological impact of the disaster and provide emergency psychiatric first-aid. Short-term planning included the following:

A. Armenia:

1. Coordinating the dispatch to Armenia of teams of Armenian-speaking mental health professionals from the U.S., Canada and Europe was necessary to provide direct patient care. Fluency in the Armenian language, some knowledge of the culture, and emotional stability were key criteria in the selection of the volunteers. Based on the author's experience, those without a knowledge of the language and culture arrived at erroneous conclusions in their assessments of the survivors' mental health and further drained the limited resources of the community by requiring translators. Though the surviving community was fluent in Armenian and Russian, only about twenty percent of the university graduates had a working knowledge of the English language.

2. Each interdisciplinary team included a psychiatrist, a psychologist, and a psychiatric nurse or psychiatric social worker. Interdisciplinary groups were helpful in many ways. First and foremost, they were to be role models for the professionals in Armenia, where not only did the psychiatrists and psychologists not work together, but they were also supervised by different government ministries. Psychiatry was supervised by the Ministry of Health and Psychology supervised by the Ministry of Education. Psychologists were not permitted to care for patients and there were no psychiatric nurses or social workers in Armenia. There were a handful of psychotherapists in Yerevan who were psychiatrists with a year of post-psychiatry training, which frequently took place in Moscow or Leningrad. Each mental health outreach team remained in Armenia for 15-22 days and provided services at the major disaster sites.

3. Each team was also joined by a psychiatrist and a psychologist from Armenia for the purposes of training, education and role modeling. This was a successful attempt at involving and empowering the survivor community. This integration also enhanced the sharing of a variety of theoretical perspectives and clinical interventions. The author encouraged the involvement of Soviet mental health professionals from other republics as well. As a result, scholars from Moscow and Georgia joined in the collaborative research effort.

4. Orientation sessions and workshops in the United States were organized for the volunteer professionals who agreed to serve in Armenia. These sessions were designed to inform, educate and empower the volunteers. This was done through a step-by-step plan.

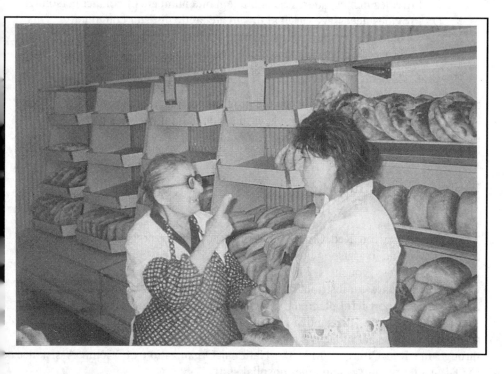

Four months hence: Dr. Anie Sanentz Kalayjian in Spitak Armenia
April 1989
Short-term planning phase of the Mental Health Outreach to Armenia

Disaster Volunteer Training Orientation

A. Provides a review of disaster literature, placing emphasis on common psychological symptomatology post-disasters.

B. Provides the findings of the initial assessment.

C. Provides names, addresses and telephone numbers of contact personnel.

D. Provides necessary survival tips in a chaotic disaster community. This includes personal items to bring such as clothing and food, items to bring for others, such as gifts, and things needed for the volunteer outreach work, including crayons, paper, pens and pencils.

5. In addition, there was a coordinated program to channel much-needed medication, educational materials, articles on natural disasters and general medical supplies to the surviving community.

B. Florida After Hurricane Andrew:

The American Red Cross, the FEMA and other organizations were very active and visible in assisting hurricane survivors. There were long lines formed to obtain Red Cross vouchers for household items, clothing and other supplies. Countless meals were distributed as Red Cross trucks drove through the streets. As part of the short-term planning, the U.S. military had established tent cities for shelter; these were dismantled when FEMA provided trailers to qualified applicants. Some additional psychological and spiritual counseling was provided through the Red Cross, FEMA, the National Organization of Victim Assistance (NOVA), clergy, nurses and other hospital staff.

The Red Cross expenditure was estimated at $77 million, with 12,150 workers serving over 4.78 million meals and providing 16,565 medical treatments. The Red Cross also established 230 shelters in Southern Florida, housing 85,154 people.

According to FEMA, there was a total of 184,893 total applications, including 46,982 families who requested assistance. As part of short-term planning, home loans for 17,511 were approved for $389 million and 5,097 small business loans were approved for $226 million. Emergency grants of 66,590 were approved for $187 million, of which 61,616 families received emergency food stamps totaling $25.8 million; 7,236 disaster unemployment claims were submitted totaling over $12.4 million.

C. Southern California After Earthquake, 1994:

As part of the short-term planning, the American Red Cross assisted both by sending volunteers and employees as well as establishing shelters for the survivors. A team of over 15,000 trained ARC relief workers, including 122 volunteers and employees from New York State, went there to meet the emergency needs of the earthquake's survivors. Over 22,000 people stayed in 47 Red Cross shelters and were served about 1.7 million meals. This operation cost the ARC over $37 million.

The immediate physical needs of the survivors were met with food, shelter and clothing, while the emotional needs were also met by trained Red Cross mental health nurses and counselors, as well as other groups of mental health professionals from California. According to Warren Zorek, chairman of Disaster Services for ARC/NY and among the first group of volunteers who rushed to the West Coast, "Some people were afraid to go back to their homes, even though their homes were unaffected by the quake." Zorek stated he heard stories regarding survival that he had never heard before, even from those he had helped following Hurricane Andrew in 1992 and Hurricane Hugo in 1989.

Eighteen Red Cross service centers opened in the Los Angeles area immediately after the quake. Caseworkers assigned there met individually with families to discuss their unique needs as a result of the quake.

The Clinton administration and other companies and organizations also participated in the short-term planning after the 1994 earthquake in southern California. Within two days after the earthquake, Southern California Edison Co. (SCE) had restored electric service to nearly all of its 1.1 million customers who had lost power and by January 23, 1994, Southern California Gas Co. had repaired all damaged lines. On January 25, 1994, the Clinton administration announced a $7.5 billion aid package, which included $6.6 billion in new federal spending plus $897 million in already released contingency funds. FEMA received the largest amount of the money, $3.9 billion, including $408 million previously committed. The Federal Highway Administration received $1.35 billion, on top of the $41 million previously received. These funds were instrumental in assisting the surviving community to re-establish its equilibrium.

Other private companies, including a number of advertising agencies in Los Angeles, launched collection drives to help their employees who had sustained damage or loss in the devastating earthquake, thus assisting in the short-term planning phase of the recovery amid the mental and physical aftershocks.

As part of the short-term planning of the outreach effort from Armenia a collaborative plan was established between hospitals in the U.S. and Armenia. The plan was designed to address the emergency physical needs of the survivors. In the planning section, Haikaz Grigorian, MD, describes a typical hospital collaborative effort.

Hospital Collaborative Efforts

Haikaz Grigorian, MD

The following is a description of some trials and tribulations experienced in the care of fifty Soviet Armenians injured during the December 7, 1988 earthquake in Armenia. These patients were brought to the tri-state hospitals of New York, New Jersey and Connecticut for specialized surgery after their initial emergency treatment and surgery in Soviet Armenian hospitals.

The first group of seven patients sponsored by Americare was treated at the joint Disease Hospital in New York City. Subsequently, more than forty patients arrived sponsored by the Armenian General Benevolent Union (AGBU) and Medical Outreach to Armenia to be treated in fifteen different hospitals in New Jersey, New York and Connecticut.

This author was asked to chair the Medical Board and a committee of Armenian-American mental health professionals, and traveled to Soviet Armenia shortly after the earthquake to assess the extent of the disaster. After a tour of the earthquake zone in the capital Yerevan, an opportunity arose to assist Project Hope surgeons who were selecting patients to be brought to Boston, Philadelphia, Chicago and Virginia hospitals for treatment. These observations led to the conclusion that these patients, during and after their medical and surgical treatments, would also need mental health counseling and support. The following is a brief summary of that experience. There are three components: patients, caretakers and volunteers.

A. Characteristics of the patients

1. Age

Sensitivity to the needs of the children as opposed to the needs of adolescents, young adults and adults was essential. This was apparent in the case of children who had a parent or parent surrogate accompanying them on their journey as was done by Project Hope, as opposed to children who were brought without parents. Project Hope had duplicated what was customary in Armenia, in that a member of the family always stays in the hospital with the child. This facilitated decision-making and the children generally felt more secure. On the other hand, those children and adolescents brought by Medical Outreach, AGBU and Americare, were not accompanied by significant others, so their caretaker volunteers became parent surrogates.

Children who were orphaned by the earthquake needed special sensitivity. Some did not know that they had lost one parent or both parents and knowing when to tell them and how to tell them was a challenge to the caretakers.

The adolescents and young adults presented concerns about the changes in their bodies and how they would fare after their return to Armenia in their social and career relationships. One young adult, a piano student with hand and foot injuries, was anxious as well as angry about her inability to pursue a career in music.

The adults had a great deal of mourning to do about losses of family members and friends, and expressed occupational preoccupation's. Three of them began to write poetry to vent their sorrow and grief. One 28-year-old woman, who had lost 2 children and a 6-month pregnancy, was a special challenge, after her left leg amputation.

2. Hospitalization

Even under the most normal circumstances hospitalization is a drastic change in a patient's life. The patients we saw in the United States had been hospitalized from the beginning of the earthquake and had undergone emergency surgery under the most dire circumstances. They were showing symptoms of Post-traumatic stress response such as screaming upon the sight of blood or syringes. They had flashbacks, were unable to sleep and refused to eat. Some of the volunteers, not having previously seen such behavior, became extremely anxious and sought consultation with the Armenian mental health professionals. The Armenian mental health professionals also began to feel the stress and strain, also never having experienced a similar situation. This author was elected to chair the clinical conferences, which were held weekly, to discuss the condition of the patients. Each member of the team was assigned to meet with a patient regularly. This became a training ground for some who later became volunteers for psychiatric outreach programs in the earthquake zone in Armenia. Later in March and April, with a much larger group in New Jersey, New York and Connecticut, this author was asked to chair the medical board. Regular meetings with the Board and special meetings with the volunteers were helpful.

3. Beliefs

The beliefs of the patients and language differences were also barriers, in that it is customary for clergy in the United States to visit the sick at hospitals. Clergy from all the Armenian churches, Apostolic, Protestant and Catholic, visited the patients and gave each one of them a Bible in Armenian. The assumption was that these patients had been exposed to religious education. The majority of the patients did not have the slightest idea about Christianity or the Armenian Church. Obviously there had been a gross under-estimation of the influence of the Soviet atheist government on its citizens. Perhaps this was denial on the part of the clergy. Only during funerals had some of the patients seen clergy in their native land and associated them with death. This also increased the anxiety level of the patients. Although all the mental health professionals and volunteers were somewhat proficient in conversational Armenian, patients had great difficulty understanding them. This escalated patients' level of stress.

B. Characteristics of the Caretakers

The non-Armenian physicians, surgeons and nurses who had volunteered their services in more than fifteen hospitals, approached these patients with extreme care, consideration and compassion through volunteer interpreters. Similarly, the hospital administrators whose hospitals were providing the hospital facilities without charge showed considerable understanding and patience, as some of the incidents connected with patients created administrative problems.

The group of Armenian mental health professionals included psychiatrists, psychologists, social workers and psychotherapists. None of the professionals had first hand experience caring for seriously wounded survivors of a calamity of such magnitude. It was obvious that briefing and debriefing of those professionals was necessary. However, this was an absolute emergency and an immediate response was necessary. Every Saturday morning the group gathered for both briefing and debriefing by exchanging observations and feelings. The group was also able to help the volunteers with their feelings.

C. Characteristics of the Volunteers

Normally, volunteers are trained by professionals in a hospital to help the staff and the patients. In this case, the volunteers did not have any preparation and they had to train as they continued to help.

Most of the volunteers were either immigrants or children and grandchildren of survivors of the Armenian Genocide. It was obvious that they were not able to observe the patient/volunteer boundary and they began relating to the patients as members of their families. In fact, when the patients were ready to leave the hospitals and receive ambulatory care, the volunteers took the patients into their own homes. As the patients were getting ready to return to Armenia, most volunteers had difficulty separating from them.

Understanding not only the dynamics of the individuals but also many other factors that impinged on the individual was necessary. Emphasis on the bio-psychosocial approach post-trauma in an unfamiliar environment became an essential part of the treatment and rehabilitation plan.

Finally, the caretakers and volunteers were emotionally and deeply affected by this experience, and needed special understanding and support.

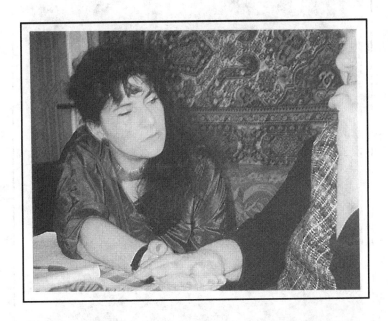

Nine months hence: Individual psychotherapy with an elderly
Armenian refugee from Azerbaijan who, having
fled the Azeri atrocities had survived the quake.

Reprinted courtesy of *The Nursing Spectrum*

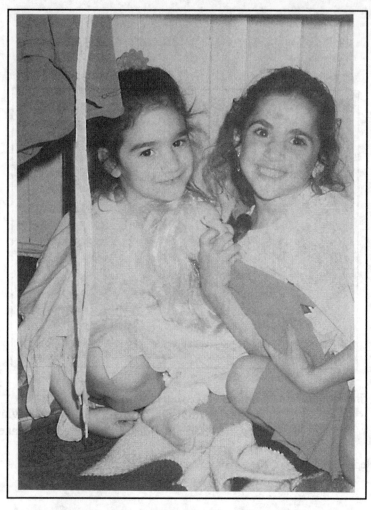

Two months hence: Post-quake play therapy session
Southern California
March 1994

Photograph by: Dr. Anie Sanentz Kalayjian

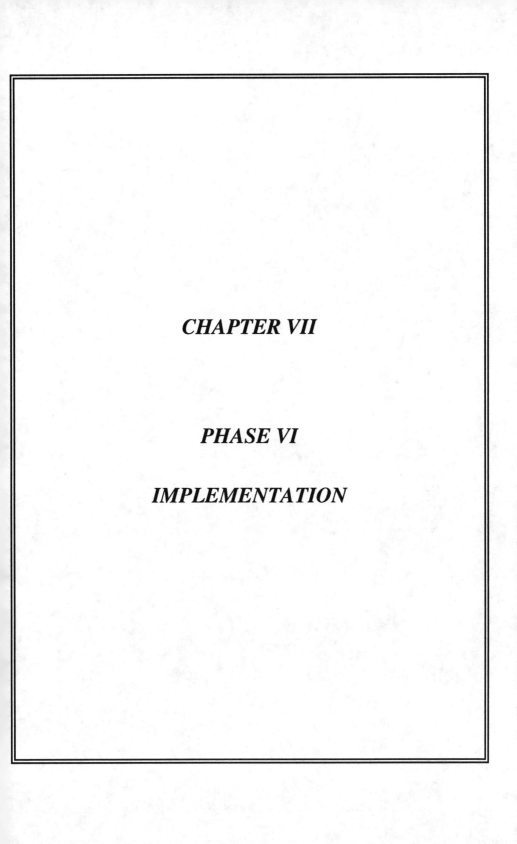

CHAPTER VII

PHASE VI

IMPLEMENTATION

CHAPTER VII

If the wrong man uses the right means,
the right means work in the wrong way.

PHASE VI

IMPLEMENTATION

Implementation is the sixth phase of MHOP. Implementation is putting the plan into effect. This phase directly follows planning, and is followed by the evaluation phase. Implementation is based on specific, unique needs of individuals and their community.

It is absolutely essential to have highly trained and expert mental health professionals conducting the interventions and implementing the plan of care. This phase may take from one month to one year based on the needs of the surviving community, their level of motivation, and resources, and number of mental health professionals available to them. Ideally, the sooner the therapeutic implementation, the sooner the community will return to its predisaster state of equilibrium.

Armenia:

The MHOP's planning phase, emphasizing the short-term goals, began in February 1989 and was re-evaluated and modified six months later, in August 1989. During this planning phase, six mental health teams went to Armenia to help the survivors of the quake, a total of forty volunteers. They helped over 3,500 earthquake survivors in Yerevan, Leninakan, Kirovakan, Spitak and in five other villages. The author, in collaboration with the President of the Committee for Cultural Relations with Armenians Abroad, Mr. Garen Dallakian, placed the volunteers in available shelters, hospitals, schools, clinics and governmental agencies to provide their professional services to a variety of people. Routine cruising, driving, or walking around was also used to detect those who, for many reasons, including fear and suspicion, did not volunteer to seek assistance. Developing a trusting relationship with the survivors was essential. The voluntary nature of the services was stressed and the benefits of the program were listed.

The mental health volunteers possessed expertise in a variety of theoretical methods, and thus clinical approaches also varied. Therapeutic techniques utilized included art therapy, biofeedback, the coloring storybook, drawings (structured and unstructured), family therapy, group therapy, instruction booklets, Logotherapy, meditation, play therapy, pharmacotherapy and short-term psychotherapy. No single clinical intervention alone would have been successful to treat all post-quake symptomatology.

Florida and California:

Implementation began immediately after Hurricane Andrew in Southern Florida and the earthquake in Southern California. No waiting period was essential to access these communities since these two natural disasters occurred in the United States.

Therapeutic Intervention Modalities

The following therapeutic intervention modalities are reviewed and summarized for their applicability in disaster communities. Some of the interventions are traditional and well-established (i.e., art therapy, group therapy, play therapy, bio-feedback and stress inoculation training); expressive art training is an ancient modality with a modern focus and also very effective in a large group. Eye Movement Desensitization and Reprocessing (EMDR) is a new modality which is still being studied. Lastly, Symbolic Expressive Therapy, another new, innovative and experimental modality is in its infancy.

Any therapeutic modality that could be done in a group format is desirable for the short-term component of the outreach program. Due to the large number of people affected by disasters, and the limited period available for effective and expeditious intervention, group methodology is preferred. The most effective modalities were: group art therapy, group play therapy, group bio-feedback and stress inoculation training, and group Logotherapy.

Art Therapy

Art therapy is a tool to facilitate the expression of feeling, and therefore, it is also a tool to facilitate healing. It is frequently the choice for treatment with children who may be too threatened to verbalize their feelings or are unable to express inner feelings. Having children and adolescents draw or paint about themselves, their families and their school or home can furnish valuable vehicles for evaluation, diagnosis and treatment.

A. Art Materials:

The choice of art materials depends highly on the setting, the child's age, dexterity and patience and the specific problem and the type of the art project itself. In general, for children under the age of four, large pieces of paper, large crayons, felt pens, finger paints and Play-Dough are recommended. On the other hand, older children may use brushes, pencils, collage materials and paper of various sizes.

B. Stages in Children's Art:

Scribbling stage: May begin at around age two and end at around four years. These scribbles usually have a specific meaning for the child and it is recommended that one speak with the child regarding the scribbles.

Preschematic stage: Begins at around age four and ends at seven. The drawings have forms and images and are more representational.

Schematic stage: Beginning at around age seven and ending at age nine. In this stage children draw the world as it appears to them; it is highly individualized.

Realistic stage: Begins at around age nine; the drawings contain more detail and are more realistic. In this stage the subject matter extends beyond the child's own immediate world.

It is recommended to ask the following questions when talking with children regarding their art work:

1. Please tell me about your drawing.

2. Where are you in this drawing?
3. Where are mommy and daddy (or other significant people for this child)?
4. Identify a theme or a feeling associated with the scribbles and ask the child's opinion.

It is recommended to use a 75-minute session, which will provide 15 minutes each for set up, discussion and clean-up and 30 minutes in project time.

Art therapy was utilized individually or in a group. Survivors were encouraged to draw, paint and form sculptures to express their feelings. Then they were encouraged to talk about their art. Some of the art work was then brought to the United States and exhibited at the Children's Museum in New York City and at various professional conferences. Art therapists were contacted in New York and Florida to assist in the analysis of the artwork brought from Armenia. This analysis was then shared with the surviving community.

Completing a piece of artwork establishes a feeling of accomplishment and pride and display of that finished product builds a sense of competency and self esteem (Metrick and Zelman, 1993). According to Kazanis (1993), an associate professor of art education at the University of Southern Florida, art helps people express and deal with their pain. She utilizes expressive art therapy with both children and adults at The Life Center, a Center for Attitudinal Healing (Tampa), and is especially interested in the power of the art-based trauma interventions as a means of prevention of later physical and mental illness, violence and substance abuse. According to Kazanis, who is the artist in residence, and Baker (1992), the Life Center's executive director, the arts provide a safe structure for children's creative expression in a time of inner chaotic feelings. Such expression is transformative and promotes healing and health.

Expressive Arts Therapy

Barbara Kazanis, EdD, CET

This section discusses the management of natural and other disasters from the point of view of the expressive arts. The expressive arts are presented within the perspective of trauma and within the intervention strategies of defusing and debriefing. The expressive arts are explored in terms of how they help:

1. To provide additional ways of working with trauma, on site, immediately afterward and with long-term Post-traumatic stress disorder. That may include visual, somatic, kinesthetic and ceremonial techniques, as well as "talking" interventions found in current intervention methods of defusing and debriefing

2. To create a larger, cognitive, framing and spiritual reforming that can encompass the catastrophic event.

3. To provide essential clarity and full expression of the experience/event.

4. To provide personal rituals and communal ceremonies to bring closure to the trauma experience.

5. To contribute to the healing of the trauma through the participatory experiential quality of the arts and directly contribute to re-establishing the essential bonding needed to heal the most severe traumatic wounding.

Models are presented for various times, kinds and levels of interventions. These include expression, assessment for at risk and healing.

The Expressive Arts: An Approach to Disaster Intervention

Introduction

No one wants to think that a disaster can really happen, but when it does, we want to know what we can do. Some who may be reading this are front-line emergency workers and volunteers. But increasingly, other professionals are seeking to contribute their specific skills in disasters. And a cadre of volunteers are involved in the creation of local civil disaster teams. The information and models presented here are intended to demonstrate the integration of the expressive arts into disaster intervention methods. They are also chosen to introduce new possibilities for the utilization of the expressive arts in order to achieve the goals of intervention and to suggest new and effective ways with which they can help in the healing process.

Trauma

For many, the experience of the disaster is traumatic. Trauma shatters our world, especially a child's world:

> "Our city is cracked,
> there was nowhere to go
> but down, lower and lower
> I am torn
> just as my city is cracked."

Child's poem from Loma Prieta Quake
(Trauma: The School's Response Video, 1991)

With natural disasters, a force beyond us moves the elements we call nature (wind, water, air and earth). Natural forces, which we usually think of as life-supporting or as creative forces, cannot be controlled or predicted. One's life will never be the same. From the point of view of the child, an adult can't fix it or find a way to guarantee that it won't happen again.

With violence, natural or man-made, there is an encounter with something beyond our understanding and often beyond our acceptance. At the most severe levels of trauma there is often more than the sorrow of great loss. There can be an assaultive quality to the unpredictable way the integrity of our order is ripped away from us. One's essential bonding with a basic trust in life can be threatened. Then one must find, not only a way to re-establish basic meaning and relationships, but also an integration of the experience into a larger order that includes this event in a meaningful way. We require rebonding to heal. No wonder the Chinese define a "crisis" as both an opportunity and a danger.

Our responses to trauma may be very intense and varied, but need to be accepted as normal responses. Equally important, the healing of trauma follows natural movements. Movement is life and life is always moving. The kind of movement referred to here is a deep organic sense of one's life being connected to the pulse of life. The shock of trauma in disasters freezes us. We stop moving.

Primary Interventions
"Moving through the event/experience"

Primary trauma interventions in disasters emphasize *"ways to move through the experience,"* usually by telling our stories. The focus of this article will be on ways to achieve this and the *"telling of our stories."* It will present and demonstrate how the arts provide channels to communicate information, express feelings and transform our views, thereby promoting healing.

Defusing/Debriefing

The primary methods utilized today to keep one "moving through the event" are called defusing and debriefing. They could be understood to focus upon "telling one's story."

Defusing is a supportive, personalized, safe, interactive process between individuals in small groups, with a facilitator providing an opportunity to develop clarity and complete expression of the event/experience. It can be emotional, include a focus on developing coping skills and encourage healing (FEMA 219 Nov. 1991, P.3).

Debriefing is a more formal, structured, planned process keyed to a group. The focus is to identify and talk about problems and issues which are related to an event. Anyone may speak. An attempt is made to bring *closure* to the event and to understand the *process* with which the person is involved.

There are several ways in which the arts and the expressive arts have or could be integrated with the methods of defusing/debriefing:

1. Talk and draw techniques.
2. Somatic techniques.
3. Kinesthetic and movement techniques for clarity and full expression.
4. Closure through personal rituals and communal ceremonies.

Defusing/Debriefing
The Talk and Draw Techniques

The primary technique utilized in defusing and debriefing has been talking about the event and sharing personal experiences. Recently, a program for the training of teachers to help children cope with disasters, developed by the Alameda County Mental Health Services with Alameda School Personal and funded by FEMA, formally introduced drawing as a primary tool to be utilized in all aspects of the defusing process, including drop-in programs for parents (Trauma: The School's Response, The Loma Prieta Earthquake Project, Video, 1991).

This program followed the essentials of defusing, moving from a general to a specific and then a personal response. It utilized leading and open-ended questions for talk/discussion and was used with drawings as "themes." The drawings were treated as a distinctive language of communication, with respect to the distinctive qualities of that language. The same care was taken as would be followed in a talk-oriented group to respect the development of self-identity through "times lines" techniques and to end with "anchoring" in a new sense of coping and empowerment.

For example, if the children drew themselves after the quake as broken, or unable to complete their faces, or heads, rather than as people who had stronger senses of their abilities to cope, a referral could be made for further assistance (Trauma: The School's Response, The Loma Prieta Earthquake Project, Video, 1991).

It is important to consider the expressive means available, and even necessary, to tell our story. Even more so, how important it is then that we take seriously the purpose and need for the telling of the story of the traumatic event in communicative forms and ways of expression appropriate to that person and to that story.

In Stockton, California, there was an individual who came into the school with an automatic weapon and injured 20 children and killed five. All of these children were Southeast Asian. While some children are taught to express their feelings, some children are taught not to feel pain, not to express pain or anger. Some are even taught you are a better person if it is not expressed. Here the question is how to engage the children, or parents, some of whom may still be struggling with English. What is needed are ways to communicate and individuals with the ability to communicate in multimodal ways (Trauma: The School's Response, The Loma Prieta Earthquake Project, Video, 1991).

In addition to "talk" and "draw" techniques, other expressive modalities may be essential for information, communication and transformation.

Defusing/Debriefing
Somatic Techniques

Earlier it was discussed that in the shock of trauma, we freeze, do not move and are unable to "tell our story" and to describe our experience. In addition, the goal of intervention methods was to *"keep one moving through the experience and to tell the story."* Thus, it is important in interventions for the management of disaster to stabilize shock and trauma physically as well as emotionally, and to understand its role in the process of cognitive framing as well as spiritual reframing.

Here the expressive arts, especially movement-based arts therapies, are a powerful way to keep one both *"moving through the experience/event"* and to unlock earlier trauma. We can become locked/immobilized at the body level and the cognitive/emotional level.

Locking on the Emotional Level:

On an emotional level we stop the movement of the event because we don't have a meaning for it, a way to move with it, or a frame of reference that carries grounding. The unexplained experiences, the images, or the event can become frozen in time. We cannot tell our story.

Locking on the Body Level:

Another way to understand this freeze that occurs in shock is *on a body level.* The breath is movement. This movement is constant both externally through the lungs and internally through cellular breath. In shock, or during prolonged stress, we take a breath in and throw our heads back a certain way, in an extreme flexion. We hold that breath in a certain way, creating a unique, functional reversal of the sensory-motor pathways. Functional as this reversal is in a moment of crisis, if we don't fully release it, images and kinesthetic-visceral responses can get locked in the nervous system, creating patterns that tend to express themselves as repetitive loops of reaction. Our story is frozen in our body. We cannot discuss our story. We may even lose consciousness of our story.

Likewise, in *"telling our story,"* the body as a language is important. In trauma management theory, the first 72 hours are assigned an essential importance for defusing and debriefing. Mitchell and Bray (1990), in their book *Emergency Services Stress*, have suggested that attending to work on a bodily level with guided imagery, breathing techniques, progressive and/or systematic relaxation techniques can be crucial in the prevention of the locking of images into and the formation of repetitive loops of response by the nervous system.

In the expressive and healing arts, there is a body-based therapy technique that has been described by Cohen (1993), a pioneer in experiential anatomy and the creator of the School for Body Mind Centering. In her training workshops and in her book, *Sensing Feeling and Action, the Experiential Anatomy of Body Mind Centering* (1993), she teaches a technique for systematic body re-education that can release the kind of sensory motor reversal in the nervous system described earlier. The technique and theory are further replicated by a professional dancer-therapist, Olsen, in her book *Body Stories*, (1993). This technique includes the practice of becoming aware through image or sensation of all discomforts found experientially in the front torso. These are experientially "brought" around the ribs "to that segment of the spine" "they" seem to choose through a sense of a "gravitating awareness." One's attention is lightly held at the chosen spinal segment. After a short period of time, sometimes longer and seeming to coincide with a 20-minute rhythmic cycle, there is often a release of the sensory motor reversal and an indicative movement response as this reversal integrates through the autonomic nervous system. The movement signals a reversal/reintegration in the nervous system and a freeing of the sensory-motor pathways to return to their everyday state of functionality.

In this author's practice (Kazanis) as a body-based expressive arts therapist, it has become clear that the effects of this technique are not limited to the first 72 hours after trauma, but seem to be profoundly effective with long-term Post-traumatic stress as well. These techniques may be akin to the same quieting effect on the autonomous nervous system reported by the relaxation response found in silent meditation. They point us to a powerful somatic basis for trauma interventions in disaster management that has not yet fully been explored as a form of trauma therapy.

Movement

Movement is a primary medium of expression. All forms of expression begin with a movement impulse which then transforms into words, sounds, gestures, colors, lines or images. In other expressive means, our inner experience is externalized in a material other than ourselves. But in movement expression, the movement of our bodies is the instrument of expression.

Certain movements and postures can help to release and express emotions such as anger, grief, sadness, agitation and confusion. We also see this process in developmental play with children at emergency sites.

Defusing/Debriefing
Kinesthetic Techniques

In the process of *"telling our story"* and creating images and symbols for it, we are constantly trying to create a new frame of meaning. It is here that the natural movements of healing within the person reveal themselves and we get closer to developing clarity and finding complete expression of the events, which is the goal of the defusing/debriefing process.

By utilizing movement-based expression, the arts speak to us as a direct visceral experience. They do not go through the cognitive mind as words. Therefore, they reveal feeling states, self-concepts and energy levels. They reveal kinesthetic messages and are another language of the body, arising from sensations and perceptions. They bridge the inner and outer realities, not only symbolically, but actually. In the moment of doing, they engage the individuals as a single unit of action. And through the intensity of focusing during the creative act/action, it is possible to actually transform the repressed feelings into constructive energy. It is by exploring these conflicting elements that avenues for insight and integration may be created that not only represent the deeper movements of our lives at work, but are organizing them and revealing them simultaneously (Rogers, 1993).

This revelation is demonstrated in the following process technique, developed by Kazanis (1988) entitled *"Theater of the Soul."* This movement-based technique was discovered while working with the need "to tell the story" and to uncover the "inner movements" of deep and hidden grief.

Kazanis' technique allows the person to choose their own objects representing "power" and "important meanings," to arrange them in their own way, on a specially selected ground chosen by them. In the exploring and moving of the objects into an arrangement, they both reveal the dynamics of reorganization that are actually occurring deep within them, but which are not yet visible or conscious. This technique allows for a specificity and fullness, as well as a deep connection, to actual life concerns. There is an inherent safety and respect that occurs within this process. Insights are set in motion unconsciously, non-verbally and can stay on the private level or can be consciously shared as the person becomes aware of them.

There is a tremendous sense of privacy and respect involved, which should not be violated by others in a group setting. There is strong support among participants, a deep sense of community, which even when consciously acknowledged is primarily experienced in action and often remains non-verbal.

The following is an excerpt from a publication that details the depths of this expressive process and how it might work for individuals who are confronted with so much trauma that numbing and freezing dominate.

105

Theater of the Soul

What happens when we can't cry? What sense of solidity and slowness of movement, maybe even stillness, comes upon us in our mind, our body and our hearing? How do we find a safe and comforting way to allow the necessary body sensations and feelings for the tears to come? How do we find a practice that provides us with "comfort" while we are in the midst of the often tumultuous movement "from groceries and gas to the awe of the absence of one we loved?" What is that swiftness and the uncontrollable back and forth that we find happening to ourselves that seems to have a life of its own and which we want so much to control and cannot? How to find a way to acknowledge that we know we are in the presence of something at work that is "more" than just ourselves.

(Kazanis, 1991)

As a child, art seemed to be the only thing that enabled this author to express herself. So, she had long had a habit of making and collecting things. But we all collect things and arrange them in curious little spaces in our homes and offices. There is a wonderful comfort in collecting things, especially objects from nature. A long walk alone and Mother Nature seems to provide some gift, some fresh moment of connection that we simply feel. We reach for an object and bring it home. Sometimes we keep these little gifts for a very long time and find them moving with us from place to place, over and over. Each time they are to be moved, we run them over in hand and eye, mind and heart and yet pack them away once more. For some inexplicable reason, it seems we have imbued them with connections symbolizing persons, events and feelings in our life. The author had an enormous number of special little objects that had been arranged around her house in groupings. She moved them often and "played" with them. It occurred to her that they resembled small altars, the kind in which people place important remembrances, prayers, wishes, losses and the mysterious tears people either haven't shed or are now shedding and need to acknowledge - small altars where we are able to be present to deep feelings and meanings for a moment or two because we are able to focus and feel connected to something deeper and bigger than themselves, making it safe to open their hearts and really be present for the moment - small altars where things that felt solid and immovable seem spontaneously to begin to shimmer and move and a certain ease of breath comes to them. Perhaps the tears of a heart that is overflowing and in need of emptying can be expressed, allowing the quiet that comes from such tears to arise in the heart and body. The author collected some objects around and then one day took them outside and placed them on very dark rich moist earth and began to move them

106

around, trying out all the possible relationships of each object to the others, until it felt "just so." She had no idea what had been made, but knew it was right and knew it told a story-the necessary story that could find no words. It gave a sense of being able to sit "quiet" for a moment. Only when it came time to take the arrangement apart and put the objects away did she realize what was done. It was a "funeral." A special kind of funeral. And it came to her to call the arrangement "funeral for a young girl." A present loss, the death of her father, brought up not only present grief but all of this old grief as well, often leaving her confused. The arrangements done at times of need provided a safe and prayerful way to find a path through the meanings and appropriate tears. They gave her something concrete, something actual, something present. They brought the grief alive and moved it in a way that gave her a point of comfort and a sense of the safety of connectedness. The author makes arrangements whenever she feels like something is stirring and feels that she is ready to allow the movement to occur. Many times she only has a sense of what is happening but that doesn't seem to really matter. Somehow making the arrangement moves her sense of emptiness, darkness or despair and when she feels the movement she somehow feel alive again and that is when she can cry. Only then does it seem that she is in the presence of truth in a direct way that is bearable in her heart no matter how painful it is. And only then, she feels comforted and bonded with life in a larger way (Kazanis, 1991).

Kazanis used this method with groups as large as 25 people or individually in private sessions and trained many other therapists to use the method. It was especially effective in working with the survivors of suicide where patterns of meanings were so difficult to come to terms with or understand. The results consistently demonstrated that previously unexpressed grief was released. Tears, previously unshed, came forth. Over and over, healing moments arose out of this contact with deep patterns of meaning and connection for the person from within, and in their own lives.

After disasters, this technique is applied to moments when one must organize those few objects of import which may have been saved or to help individuals determine what and how to reconstruct what has been saved after their immense losses. In a natural disaster, this process may be of therapeutic benefit to arrive at both clarity and completeness of expression and a deeper sense of the internal movements of meaning and re-organization at work within the person.

In another story of the expressive arts, Joan Borysenko, a psychologist who works in the field of psychoneuroimmunology, tells the story of a therapist working in shelters for battered women where the women have only 30 days to re-ground and reestablish themselves before they must return to the community. She notes that, in addition to the traditional talk therapies and techniques of empowerment, the single most effective tool of reconnection to help the women ground quickly for their return to the community was the utilization of the theater and music from the women's own ethnic cultures (Boryesenko, 1993).

Documented in a profoundly touching article in *Newsweek* even in the midst of active war Sarajevans kept producing culture in nights illuminated by candles and kept warm with crude wood stoves distributed by the Red Cross and other relief agencies. According to the *Newsweek* article, the fruits of an enduring intellectual life were experienced: a film series in New York, a new play in London, a Children's Art exhibit at the Pompidou Center in Paris and the publication of a diary by a young woman (*Newsweek*, 1994).

These two stories together demonstrate the grounding capacities and the transformative qualities of the arts-even in the midst of chaos and ugliness, to create order and even manifest beauty.

Defusing/Debriefing
From Personal Rituals to Communal Ceremonies

In defusing and debriefing methods noted earlier there is an effort to arrive at a sense of empowerment and completion. When done with formal intention, rituals and ceremonies emerge. The act of making the ritual becomes healing in itself. The defusing/debriefing process seems to require that there be closure in both meaning and action. In instances of the deepest wounding through tragedies and disaster, closure of both meaning and action are required for the person or community to go on. It is through ceremony then, that we can hope to heal and re-establish the essential bonding that may have been wounded by the most severe trauma.

Emergency workers at the recent earthquakes in the Los Angles area have said that American-Indian victims seemed to demonstrate less evidence of trauma because the tribal medicine men and elders immediately came to Los Angeles and created rituals and ceremonies and performed traditional songs and dances to reaffirm for their people the individual and communal relationships to nature. Thus, meaning and action were reestablished and reaffirmed a basic relationship at the core of their native American beliefs (Bloch, 1994). The arts, when done with intention, as sacred, join with the ancient tradition of ceremonies and rituals through which individuals and communities have reclaimed their wholeness and expressed their vital spirit throughout history.

One of the major roadblocks to establishing this harmony in the midst of assaultive chaos is that many individuals have abandoned the traditions that in the past gave the opportunity to publicly share tragedies and grief. As a result, has been less and less permission to express it and to be supported by the community.

Ceremony at Rocky Point

One of the most touching, spontaneous examples of this process of closure by ceremony came from a tragedy at Rocky Point, a business complex in Tampa, Florida. A former employee, who had been fired, returned to the cafeteria, which had previously been established as a unique place of familial rapport and trust during the lunch hour. Here, in the presence of about 40 people, he shot five of his former bosses and killed three of them. Later, and elsewhere, he shot and killed himself. People were devastated, not only by the event, but additionally by the violation of these deaths on what had been a unique place of warmth and trust.

The University of Southern Florida's (Tampa, Florida) community psychiatric crisis intervention teams worked on-site for a week with individuals and groups, not only from that particular firm, but also with other employees in the building. At the end of the crisis intervention week, people indicated the need for a ceremony to create a closure for this horrific event.

The building administration requested that the ceremony not be funereal, but be carefully planned to help bring the requested closure. A ceremony was planned and 800 people from the entire building were invited. Over 350 people came. The administration had decided that a tree would be planted in the garden adjacent to the cafeteria. Sheryle Baker (Director of the Life Center) and Kazanis asked that large, black, Spanish garden stones be brought in for the ceremony, the kind that fit in ones hand just so, and which, when held and turned over and over, become shiny from the oils in the hand. They were offered to all who attended. A large container of these stones was placed on the site and near the newly planted tree. At the opening of the ceremony, everyone was given the opportunity to select a stone, and hold these stones as an "anchor" throughout the ceremony. There is a long and ancient tradition found in various ethnic and cultural traditions for the meaning and power of stones to be both a representation of that which is unchanging and also a reminder of one's tribal connection. It has also been used as a marker to be left indicating the deceased had been visited.

In the first part of the ceremony, individuals were asked to place *into* their stone, *to imbue it with,* any unfinished and/or all thoughts and feelings they wished to convey and/or leave at the site. In a second part of the ceremony, a formal recognition was made that there had been a rip or tear in the fiber of the community, and that not only individuals needed to feel healed, but the "place" needed to be healed, that a basic trust in the community needed to be reaffirmed as well. It was acknowledged that the communal holding of the breath needed to be released, at which point there was a palpable and auditory release, and that individuals needed to be able to acknowledge and reaffirm that there was a basic human trust between people, between them, large enough to contain such a rip in its fiber without destroying it. They affirmed that they could look each other in the eye and say, "hello, how are you?"

As a final act of completion, attendees were invited to place these stones, whenever it felt appropriate to them, at the foot of the specially planted tree. Finally, a special celebration of sharing food was held in the cafeteria, their favored place and where the event had occurred. Of remarkable impact is that when the author returned three weeks later, over 100 new black stones had been placed under that memorial tree. The ceremony had lived on.

In summary, it can be noted that, when done with formal intention, rituals and ceremonies emerge. Like the ceremony at Rocky Point, the "actual act of making" is as important as what is expressed. The art of making the ceremony is healing in itself. These kinds of expressions bring not only structure, but carry forth meaning and value.

Model Programs and Model Interventions

The following is a selected list of models which present different organizational structures and kinds of expressive arts-based interventions that can be implemented during a traumatic event and immediately after.

A. Cooperative Disaster Child Care Program - *"Listen to the Children"*

This is a service administered by the Church of the Brethren General Board in cooperation with the American Red Cross and FEMA Directed by Lydia H. Walker, this group provided child care, on site, in the immediate area where parents are filling out forms for essential services. Trained at intensive workshops held throughout the country, volunteers travel to work as needed in disaster areas and emergencies.

An area is set up where the children may stay for a short time within sight of their parents. The goal is to normalize the situation and the children. Developmentally-based, the activities center upon play and the arts. They include puppets, visual arts, music and movement. Although most children experience the simple comforts and soothing effects of playful, age-appropriate activities and benefit from a momentary sense of order in the midst of confusion, there are some profound examples of transformation that demonstrate the immediate release of trauma. One example was a child who had not talked since Hurricane Andrew and whom people were already beginning to treat as speechless, who with the help of the puppets was able to tell the essential details of her "story" and release the trauma through this expression and find her speech.

B. Trauma: The School's Response:

Trauma: The School's Response is a video created by the Loma Prieta Earthquake Project. The project and the video were funded by the Federal Emergency Management Agency (FEMA), through the National Institute for Mental Health and administered by the California Department of Mental Health. The video presents a program for mental health professionals, school administrators and teachers. Trauma's impact on children and schools, normal and prolonged stress responses, assessment considerations and intervention models are presented. It is a strong and effective graphic presentation.

A workbook, entitled *How to Help Children After a Disaster* (FEMA 219/November, 1991), created by the Alameda County Mental Health Department in conjunction with FEMA, serves as a resource for the classroom teacher in helping children to recover from the effects of a disaster. An important feature is the presentation of the general principles of defusing/debriefing for a natural disaster in terms of both **"Talk and Draw Methods."** The two methods are presented in parallel so the instructions for the utilization of the arts are clear and easily applied.

An additional workbook, created by FEMA and the Santa Cruz County Mental Health Services, entitled *School Intervention Following a Critical Incident*, was part of **Project COPE** (FEMA 220/November 1991). This was a federally-funded crisis counseling program activated in Santa Cruz, California, in response to the October 17, 1989 Loma Prieta earthquake. The project provided individual, family and group counseling, agency debriefing services and a school intervention program.

Primarily a demonstration of school debriefing using art, it includes group process, identifying children at risk, crisis management, outreach and reassurance. The methods present specific expressive arts techniques for use by the classroom teacher for expression, assessment of children at risk, and interventions. It also includes a **"Gain and Loss"** collage for the anniversary of the event. The inclusion of family drop-in programs, art-based as well as talk-based, are also included. All three of these resources are interwoven and are available upon request from FEMA.

C. The Bay Area Arts Relief Project

An example of a collaborative community response was to the Oakland area fires. "These fires had started as a brush fire on an Oakland hillside and turned into a massive firestorm. The blaze raged for more than 15 hours, destroying close to 3,000 homes and killing 25 people in a 1.99-acre stretch across the Oakland and Berkeley Hills" (Metrick & Zelman, 1992. p.7). The relief project demonstrates how the arts and expressive arts therapies can be tools for responding to a major community crisis, and how the arts can play an important and effective role in mental health strategies following a disaster in a community.

Within 24 hours of the massive firestorm, a number of arts groups mobilized to conceive an expressive arts therapy program for children in schools affected by the fire. Within five weeks, more than 100 artists and therapists working together in teams of artists/therapists entered six schools with 25 projects, based upon a variety of visual, literary and performing arts, for more than 500 students aged five to thirteen (Metrick, Zelman, 1992).

In the demonstration book entitled *Art from Ashes*, (Metrick & Zelman, 1992) many of the individual arts projects are presented and described. Both therapeutic and expressive goals as well as candidly honest evaluative outcomes are stated. The range of the teams as well as the variety of the art experiences is noteworthy and valuable. In addition, the role of the arts - in crisis intervention, the resolution of trauma, and delayed stress are discussed. The book includes extremely helpful materials on their experience in organizing as well as with funding the project. This book presentation is very thorough and meant to inspire and support the formation of local projects and teams.

D. Trauma Intervention Project for War-Afflicted Children in Croatia, Bosnia-Herzegovina and Slovenia

The most extensive trauma intervention project for war-afflicted children in Croatia, Bosnia-Herzegovina, and Slovenia, is currently being conducted under the direction of Arpad Barath, PhD, from the University of Zagreb. (Earlier sponsorship included the Croatian government and UNICEF Zagreb).

Psychologists from Croatia expressed an interest in international peer consultation and support. Ellen Bloch, PhD, Director of The Center for Trauma Intervention and Education responded. Bloch and colleagues who had been working on developing a public health model of intervention in communities impacted by the Gulf War, began a collaborative exchange with Barath who was developing an expressive arts based interventive/preventive psychosocial intervention and treatment program for the children in the Balkans, many of whom showed symptoms of PTSD. Their model, co-joined with Barath's expressive arts based program, may be very effective as an international model applied to catastrophic events and natural disasters, as well as the catastrophic effects of prolonged threats of violence and life, and long term disruption of communities.

The centerpiece of the Croatian project, which was later extended to Bosnia-Herzegovina, and Slovenia, is a public health model program based in the expressive arts. The children, (Croatian, Muslim and Serbian, ages six to fourteen) many of whom endured traumatic stress disorders, depression, anxiety, separation and loss, nightmares and family upheaval, and some of the effects of torture are being reached through a model expressive arts program. In addition to training workshops for health professionals and art teachers and the dissemination of trauma prevention information through the media, the first phase of this program, a crisis intervention experiential program, moves each child through seven expressive stages of images of life before the war, fear and anger felt during the war, and finally expression of hope, love and "messages to the world" through paintings and poetry (Bloch, 1994 p8). Each of the seven steps included: a guided relaxation tape, a selected piece of music, an artist's painting for inspiration, sometimes movement, and always a drawing exercise. The second phase of the intervention/prevention program was created to deal with secondary and longer term effects of trauma. It included a self-help and art therapy program based on the "12 steps" program we are familiar with in the U.S. A third phase that works with the integration of the community was initiated in the Fall of 1995 and includes the creation of expressive arts trauma rooms in libraries, public buildings and community centers (Barath, 1994).

Bloch brought children's art work from this program to the U.S. for the purpose of creating an exhibition which would serve to disseminate information on this program. A traveling exhibition of the children's art work form phase one: the crisis intervention program, entitled Children of War, My Childhood in Croatia was curated by Kazanis, Director of the Center for Arts and Community, USF, with the express educational, moral and aesthetic purpose of creating a visual demonstration of the actual program which would also serve as a teaching tool for the potential application of the Balkan program to local communities. The exhibition was first presented at the Tampa Museum of Art in January, 1995. It is available for travel to other sites through the Center for Arts and Community.

E. Individual Professionals and Expressive Arts Training

There are many professional therapists and expressive arts therapists who work with individuals who experienced not only natural disasters but with many kinds of trauma and Post-traumatic syndrome. There are many individuals who seek professional help in an area where a disaster has occurred, or could occur. Many therapists serve on county or school crisis teams and see, in addition to disasters, the trauma of violence which has broken out or occurs daily as part of ones community or school life. Many seek to educate or help individuals for whom past assaultive events have occurred or are carried with them from their past in other countries. Many professionals are asked to be helpers in the healing of trauma for those whose memories are thought to be left behind but find them resurfacing, waiting to be released and integrated. They have been instrumental in creating techniques and methods that are very powerful and effective with trauma that can help us to further understand the nature and healing of trauma in natural disasters.

Bio-feedback and Stress Inoculation Training

Bio-feedback (the use of instruments to become aware of minute changes in the physiological processes in the body) and Stress Inoculation Training (SIT) have also been used. The individual is usually not aware of small physiological changes within the self without training. Bio-feedback instruments provide immediate information about changes in muscle tension, skin surface temperature, skin conductivity and other physiological measures. With the use of bio-feedback instruments, individuals suffering from PTSD can identify the level of stress in their bodies. Then, with the use of appropriate relaxation techniques, they can easily monitor the progress of their relaxation training with the visual or auditory cues provided by the instruments.

Stress Inoculation Training is a treatment paradigm consisting of specific training operations combining elements of education, relaxation training, bio-feedback, imaginal desensitization, coping skills training, guided self-dialogue and real-life desensitization. About eighteen months after the quake in Armenia, SIT was utilized by Gergerian (1991) for the treatment of 115 school-age children in Leninakan who exhibited the following symptoms of PTSD: fear, somatization, sadness, forgetfulness, distractibility and lack of concentration.

Subjects were asked to list their complaints on a sheet of paper and rate each complaint on a scale of zero to ten (no complaint to severe complaint). During the first week, they were involved in the daily practice of the following relaxation techniques: progressive relaxation, yoga stretching, breathing re-training, somatic focusing, sensation scanning, somatic imagery training and meditation. Each participant used a bio-feedback stress-check card using skin surface temperature to provide visual cues as to their level of tension/relaxation prior to each training session. During the second and third week, each class participated in educational and emotional discussion groups, imaginal desensitization, coping skills training, guided self-dialogue and real life desensitization. According to Gergerian (1991), significant symptomatic improvements resulted after 10-12 intensive daily sessions of SIT during a three week period. The preliminary findings revealed an over fifty percent (50%) decrease in symptoms such as fear, somatic pains and sadness, and an over 80% improvement in memory and concentration.

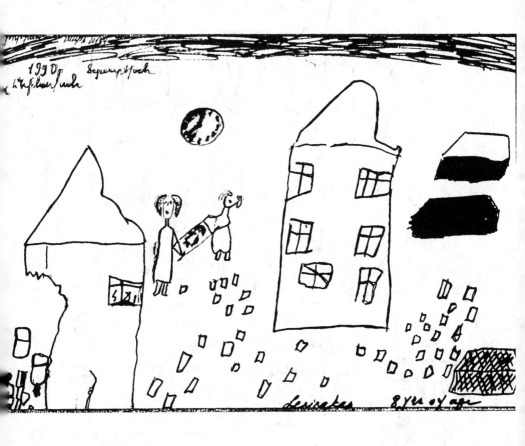

Three weeks hence: An eight-year-old Armenian girl from
Leninakan, Armenia depicting her rescue
efforts during the earthquake.
January, 1989

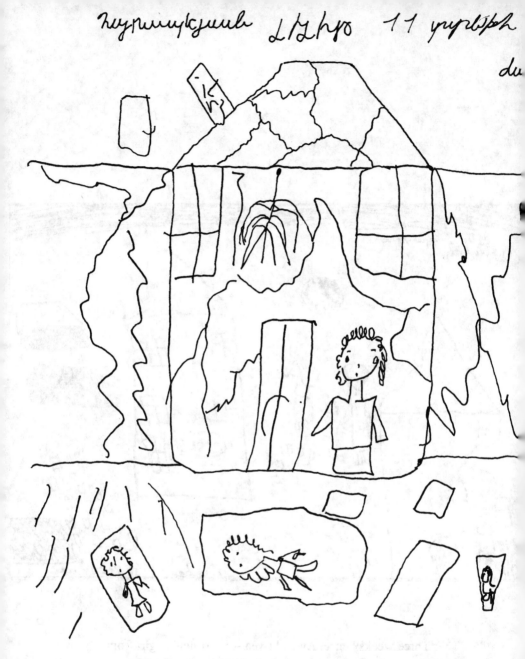

Three weeks hence: An eleven-year-old girl from Leninakan,
Armenia commits to paper her impressions
of the earthquake.
January, 1989

116

Eye Movement Desensitization and Reprocessing (EMDR)

Edmund L. Gergerian, MD

A new treatment method using an interactive standardized desensitization and cognitive restructuring approach in combination with the use of saccadic eye movements has been developed by Shapiro (1989a, 1989b, 1995) for the effective and accelerated reprocessing of unresolved traumatic memories in PTSD survivors. This new method is called Eye Movement Desensitization and Reprocessing (EMDR).

In the summer of 1987, Francine Shapiro was preoccupied with disturbing thoughts. She took a walk in Los Gatos park in California and noticed that her eyes moved spontaneously up and down, in a diagonal direction, repetitively, and the disturbing thoughts seemed to lose their intensity or disappear. When she attempted to voluntarily bring back the disturbing thoughts, they had lost their negative affective change and were no longer causing disturbance. EMDR evolved out of this phenomenon. Shapiro, a research psychologist at the Mental Research Institute in Palo Alto, associated the dissolution of the disturbing memories that were preoccupying her that day with the experience of spontaneous rapid eye movements. Amazed by her serendipitous discovery, she tested her hypothesis in a study using 22 subjects (Shapiro, 1989a) and obtained effective treatment results. A single EMDR session "successfully desensitized the subjects' traumatic memories and dramatically altered their cognitive assessments of the situation, effects that were maintained through the 3-month follow-up check. This therapeutic benefit was accompanied by behavioral shifts which included the alleviation of the subjects' primary presenting complaints." (Shapiro, 1989a).

Shapiro has personally trained thousands of licensed clinicians in the use of the Eye Movement Desensitization and Reprocessing treatment method and this author has also completed her training. Shapiro insists that the use of EMDR by untrained clinicians reduces the effectiveness of EMDR treatment results and puts PTSD survivors at risk. Therefore, it is important that EMDR be practiced only by trained and licensed clinicians.

Method

The following section outlines the primary components of the method, not the choice points and variations that are needed in order to arrive at a successful resolution of the target trauma. The procedures that follow are for each patient.

117

A. Subject is required to identify a disturbing image of the traumatic memory, preferably the most traumatic point in the scene or a disturbing flashback.

B. A negative cognition, an irrationally negative, self-referential belief about the memory is elicited. Patient is asked, "What words about yourself or the incident best go with the picture?," "It was my fault," "I have no control." Negative cognition's should have an effective resonance.

C. Subject is then required to elicit a positive cognition, a preferred belief statement. They are asked how they would prefer to feel. Examples of such positive self-statements include, "I did the best I could," "It's over," "I have control." This is rated by the patient on the seven point Validity of Cognition Scale, a semantic differential scale; 1=completely untrue 7=completely true(believable) (Shapiro, 1989a).

D. Subject is asked to identify emotions and body sensations that are associated with the traumatic memory and identify location(s) of body sensations.

E. Subject is asked to self-assess the traumatic memory, negative cognition, emotions and body sensations on a 11-point Subject Units of Discomfort Scale (SUDS, Wolpe, 1982) with o=no anxiety or disturbance; 10=highest anxiety or disturbance.

F. Additional instructions are given to the subject prior to the initial set of eye movements (Shapiro 1989b, 1992, 1993, 1995).

G. The patient is asked to:
(i)   visualize the memory
(ii) attend to the negative cognition, "I am out of control"
(iii) Concentrate on the physical sensations and negative emotional experience of the traumatic memory
(iv) Visually track the clinician's index and middle fingers, which are rapidly and rhythmically moved back and forth across the line of vision from the extreme right to extreme left at a 12-14 inch distance from the subjects

118

face, two back-and-forth movements per second. The back and forth movement of the clinician's fingers is repeated 12-25 times, each such grouping defined as one set.

H. After each set of saccade, the subject is instructed to "blank out the picture and take a deep breath." Then, subject is asked, "What comes up for you?" or "What are you noticing now?" or "What do you get now?" Periodically, a SUDS rating is obtained.

I. When the SUDS levels reaches 'O' or '1' the positive desired cognition is tested by asking, "How do you feel about (the positive cognition) from 1-7?", "How true and believable does it feel?"

J. When the positive cognition reaches '6' or '7' and the SUDS level reaches '0' or '1' the subject is asked to focus on the traumatic experience, picture or memory and concentrate on the positive cognitive. Another set of eye movements is performed to install the positive cognition.

K. A body scan, while holding the traumatic picture in mind, is done to reprocess any remaining negative body sensation.

Applications

EMDR has been used in the treatment of PTSD related to various kinds of stressors:

1. Natural disasters, such as floods, hurricanes, tornadoes and earthquakes
2. Accidental man-made disasters such as industrial accidents, auto-accidents, plane crashes, fires and;
3. Deliberate man-made disasters such as rapes, incest's, kidnapping, military combat, torture, bombings.

Grainger (1992) reported on a three-person disaster response team of EMDR-trained therapists who worked with Hurricane Andrew disaster survivors, utilizing EMDR. Pre-EMDR and post-EMDR SUDS levels were obtained on 16 survivors, the pre-SUDS averaging 8.0 and the post-SUDS averaging 2.2. Boore

(1992) reported on a larger team of EMDR-trained clinicians who also worked with Hurricane Andrew disaster survivors. Beginning and ending SUDS levels were taken. Mean SUDS level declined from 8.2 to 1.4 (n=64).

The effective use of EMDR will be illustrated through treatment of two PTSD survivors. The first patient was a survivor of the earthquake in Armenia who lost her husband during the earthquake and the second patient attempted to rescue her father who was covered with rubble following the collapse of a defective house five years after the 1988 quake. The first patient's responses have been included while most of the therapist's instructions and interventions have been omitted.

Patient A:

Traumatic memories/pictures: Earthquake pictures. "As soon as I came I saw the school building destroyed" (her husband worked as a teacher). "My son was alive at the school in a different building." Picture of dead husband, buried.

Negative Cognition: "My son has no father, I remained alone, I can't accept that."
Positive Cognition: "I can accept that my son has no father and that I am alone."
Validity of Cognition: 1
Emotion: "I would like to cry."
Location of body sensation: Headache, body weakness.
Pre-EMDR SUDs level: 8

During EMDR sets of eye movements ranged from 25 to 30 eye movements per set. Verbal responses after each set were as follows:

Set 1: "I would like to cry. My heart is beating fast."
Set 2: "I don't want to talk."
Set 3: "Nothing."
Set 4: "I was thinking about my son."
Set 5: "All of them, many of them are like my son, and like me, I am not the only one alone."
Set 6: "I am trying to remember the picture but I can't."
Set 7: "I don't know. I can't remember anything in my head. I don't want to talk."
Set 8: "I am thinking about my son. He'll grow up and I'll not be alone."

Set 9: "I don't know. I want to cry against my will."
Set 10: "I don't feel like crying ... I think that this is the way life is."
Set 11: "There are many people like me, and there are people like me."
SUDs level: 1
Validity of Cognition: 6
Set 12: Installation of Positive Cognition.

During the debriefing, patient stated that prior to the EMDR session she thought that she was the only mother that was alone. During the course of EMDR her traumatic experiences were rapidly and effectively reprocessed and she was able to realize toward the conclusion of the EMDR that there were many others like her. She was also able to see her son grow during the reprocessing, and therefore, she would not be alone, a perception not available to her prior to the EMDR.

Patient B:

Traumatic Memories/Pictures: "While talking with my sister, there was a loud noise and the room fell. I heard my father saying, "Help me!" I jumped into the rubble and asked my father. "Where are you?" I saw blood on his forehead as I moved the rubble. I held my father's head and started to cry. My mother fainted.

Negative Cognition: "I have bad luck."
Positive Cognition: "It's over, it's in the past."
Validity of Cognition: 2
Emotion: Guilt. Sorrow.
Location of body sensation: My heart hurts, shortness of breath, my whole body, headache, neck pain, flashes in my eyes and my brain.
Pre-EMDR SUDs level: 7

This patient displayed very intense abreaction's during the EMDR session. She was re-experiencing the entire event. As the building collapsed she was surrounded by dust and she started suffocating. She was about to vomit as she interrupted the eye movements and closed her eyes. The therapist firmly redirected her to open her eyes and continue the eye movements, thereby accelerating the reprocessing of the traumatic memory and preventing the vomiting. A transparent curtain appeared, separating her from the picture. Finally, the picture disappeared and the patient looked around her, loudly exclaiming in disbelief, "It's gone, it's gone! I don't see it," and started laughing out of joy. She could not bring back the memory or visualize the traumatic picture after the EMDR session.

Following the traumatic incident, the patient used to wake up with nightmares of the traumatic scene at least once a week. Nightmares of the incident stopped after one EMDR session.

Conclusion:

EMDR is a new treatment method that is both rapid and effective. EMDR could be used in all cases of PTSD. However, it requires good clinical skills, experience and formal training in EMDR.

Group Therapy

Group therapy has been utilized effectively with survivors of both the Nazi Holocaust and the Ottoman Turkish Genocide of the Armenians. According to Danieli (1980), Holocaust survivors recognize that a group offers a place for catharsis and a place to name, verbalize and express feelings. This author has found group therapy to be an effective clinical modality in working with Vietnam veterans and incest survivors, also.

Group therapy has many advantages over individual therapy. One major difference is the presence of many people with a therapist. Other differences include: receiving feedback from multiple sources, providing stimuli from multiple sources, providing an interpersonal testing ground, or trial base for new and old ways of relating to people, and coping with interpersonal issues.

According to Yalom (1975), there are eleven interdependent curative factors in group therapy that are therapeutic to the participants. These factors are the framework for an effective approach to therapy. Among the curative factors which were found to be therapeutic in natural disaster survivor groups are universality, instilling of hope and altruism.

The use of group therapy was instrumental in providing a warm, supportive and therapeutic environment for many of the survivors in Armenia, southern California and southern Florida. The survivor community expressed comfort and trust in a group setting because they were too curious and impatient with a limited concept of individual privacy to benefit from individual therapy. A mother's group, grieving group, teachers' group, poetry reading group and religious group were some of the groups developed in the survivor community. The sharing of feelings with others, being supportive to others, focusing on someone other than oneself, networking and increasing one's resources were positive effects of group participation.

It is recommended that post-natural disaster groups meet twice a week for a six-week duration, or once a week for a fifteen week duration, with each session ranging from 60-90 minutes, depending on the group size and its members' decision.

Logotherapy

Logotherapy is a form of psychotherapy, individual or group, wherein the focus is placed on meanings instead of feelings as a means of understanding and resolving conflicts and emotional difficulties. This form of psychotherapy was introduced by Viktor Frankl (1969). Logotherapy is the third Viennese School of psychotherapy, the predecessors being the Freudian and Adlerian Schools.

Although there is wide misconception that Frankl introduced his theory as a longtime prisoner of the Nazi concentration camps, he had introduced the core concepts of Logotherapy before his imprisonment. But there, in the concentration camps, he was able to put his theory to use. Although his entire family, except his sister, died in the camp, Frankl was not only able to find meaning in his suffering, he was able to help many other prisoners to exercise their will to freedom. When all is taken away from one -- due to man-made or natural disasters -- Frankl asserts to focus on "the last of human freedoms" -- the ability to choose one's attitude in a given set of circumstances." This ultimate freedom is what we can exercise in any given situation, even in the worst conceivable one.

Frankl is well-known as the author of *Man's Search for Meaning* (1969), which outlines his pioneering work pertaining to treatment of PTSD, and other existential crises. In Logotherapy or existential analysis, the human will to meaning is the core for most human behavior. In his writings, Frankl (1969,1978), consistently points out that human beings readily sacrifice safety, security, and sexual needs for things that are meaningful for them. According to Frankl (1978), being human is being always directed and pointing to something or someone other than oneself: to a meaning to fulfill or another human being to encounter, a cause to serve or a person to love. Only to the extent that one is living out this self-transcendence of human existence is only truly human or does one become one's true self.

According to Frankl (1978), each life situation is unique and the meaning of each situation must be unique. He asserts that therapists can never define what is or is not meaningful for individuals, meaning is often found in a self-transcendent encounter with the world. Just as people differ in their perceptions of trauma and in the ways that they cope with it, they also differ in the meanings they attribute to the same situation. Frankl points out that meanings and meaning potentials can be clouded, covered, and/or repressed due to a fear of responsibility, and reactive to trauma (1962). Such meaning repressions will ultimately lead to a meaning vacuum or existential vacuum. This vacuum is then filled by the development of some forms of anxiety, depression, substance abuse, phobias, and compulsive sexual behavior.

Frankl is the first psychiatrist who has recognized the positive outcomes from traumatic situations. The role of the therapist within Logotherapy is to help the trauma survivor discover a unique personal meaning. Therefore, transforming the trauma pain into meaningful awareness.

Although Frankl (1978) asserted that meaning is available under any condition, even the worst conceivable one, it was very difficult for this author to believe that finding meaning was possible immediately after the devastating earthquake in Armenia. It was enlightening to see how 20% of those interviewed perceived caring for others, helping one another, and receiving help from the world as being very meaningful only six weeks after the earthquake.

The survivors in Armenia talked about a modification of attitude and found meaning through an acceptance of blind fate. They were even convinced that they were stronger, wiser, more resourceful and more experienced for having survived the quake.

In Florida, approximately 30% of those interviewed three months after Hurricane Andrew talked about the positive meanings in their lives. Some of the survivors' responses were: "I am alive, thank God," "I was able to help my neighbor. She was all wet, her roof had caved in; mine was OK, you know," "My friend and I stayed at the street corner and guided the traffic; there were no traffic lights functioning," "Man, it was an experience, I made it through, forget my house and the material stuff, those are here today and gone tomorrow," "I know now all the petty stuff is not meaningful; there are more important things in life and God made me realize it, kind of slapped me into reality."

Play Therapy

Play therapy is another effective technique to be utilized with children, and families with young children post-natural disasters. Play therapy provides a natural atmosphere for children to express their innermost feelings, fears and anxieties.

Functions of Play:

Play has many functions. According to Wilson and Kneisel (1983), children use it to:

1. Assimilate and master past traumatic experiences that they had no control over.
2. Communicate with the unconscious.
3. Communicate with parental figures and other authority figures.
4. Explore and experiment in new ways of relating to self, others and the world.
5. Compromise between their inner drives and the outer reality.
6. Learn about self in relation to others and the world.

Setting for Play Therapy:

Ideally, play therapy needs to be done in a well-equipped playroom furnished with a variety of toys including dolls, puppets, blocks, dollhouses and furniture, cars, trucks, toy animals, musical instruments, checkers and other games. When this author utilized play therapy in Armenia as both a diagnostic tool and treatment modality, those ideal conditions were not present. The scarcity of toys stimulated creativity in the children, and they created toys from rubble, rags and pillows. Play is a natural and common activity for children wherever they may be.

Symbolic Experiential Training

Levon N. Jernazian, PhD

The core functional model of traditional therapy is the hetero-oriented, dyadic, rarely triadic setting, with a clear-cut conscious or unconscious distribution of role functions. These include that of the patient sitting and asking for help, and the therapist assisting and ultimately trying to fulfill the patient's expectations. This setting bears a conscious or unconscious shade of an inherently authoritarian, or at least an implicitly medical type of "patient-therapist" interaction, as well as reinforcement of the external motivation of the "patient."

An alternative for the traditional hetero-oriented model is provided by the self-oriented paradigm of therapy that is based upon the assumption that clients can be taught certain skills to manage their own problems individually. Some of the advantages of this approach relate to a wider range of client freedom and the development of individual coping skills. Internal orientation and self-reliance, hence personal autonomy and psychological maturity, utilization of personal achievement, motivation, and authenticity of interpersonal perception in therapeutic interaction are goals that are also ultimate tasks of hetero-oriented therapy. In hetro-oriented therapy, however, dependency and transference are eliminated. The self-oriented paradigm, however, as opposed to its hetero-oriented model, has not been developed to its full extent. The model, emerging in forms like Autogenic Training (Schultz, 1983), is either too problem-specific or designed to be secondary to other therapeutic methods. The latter dissonance between inherent possibilities of the self-oriented paradigm and its practical implementation lead to development of a wider model, *Symbolic Experiential Training (SET)*.

Theoretical and Empirical Sources

In 1986 while conducting pilot studies of collective unconscious symbols, this author approached the problem as a hard-nosed and uncompromising behavioral researcher with a well-defined structure and operational procedure. The research design consisted of the following steps:

1. Induction of a deep hypnotic trance by a standardized hypnotic technique.

127

2. Presentation of a meaningful collective unconscious single stimulus word or image in audio or visual form.
3. Free association.
4. Content-analysis of free associations of subjects from different ethno-cultural backgrounds and differentiation of cognitive-emotional patterns of reactions.

The first subject was a 34-year-old male of Armenian ethnicity. After the initial induction phase that was conducted in a permissive manner, the first stimulus word, "Eye," was presented. What follows is the abbreviated transcript of his free-associations:

"Nothing ... (heavy breathing) ... I am fully open ... My eyes are full of tears but I cannot cry ... A field, motherland, crop, dog, space. Unknown eye, one eye, one big eye, open, motionless, without eyelashes, one color, blue, very big, very ... immeasurably big eye, everything else is in the eye. I am going inside the eye. I am going and entering the eye. It is dark like in a fairy tale. They are calling, it is mysterious. I cannot go forward, but I feel. (heavy breathing) ... I am not going forward. It is black but black like a light. The blue is left behind. Lights are lit. ... The door is not opening. If I go there everything will end. ... Wait ... It seems like they are talking with me, without words, in the eye. The eye is speaking ... I do not understand (heavy, uneven breathing). The eye is breathing, I am in the eye. It is mysterious. I am asking, "what are you saying, I don't understand". He is sending waves. An ocean is opening but it's not water. It is joy, I can see mountains, immaterial ... look like people ... I want to see further, it is so close.

Seems like there is a sun in the far, black sun. It is a light night. It is safe there, safe. He says later, a long time is needed for that to open, for me to see further, very long time and I cannot see now. I am seeing only the beginning now, the point of entering. The beginning, the ocean and the mountains. To see further than that I need time, very long time. I have to stay there long enough for it to open. Maybe one century, or more, more, an eternity. It is going to be an eternity for me. And he will open. Quiet, eternity. There is not going to be time. So, something more is needed than time.

I am coming out of the eye ... I see the eye from the inside and from the outside. The lines of the eye are all mixed up ... I don't understand, I don't want to understand. I don't have to. Tears again, getting more. I don't know the reason. Again, the field.

Dog, yellow field ... I am in the air, the dog is underneath, I am hanging in the air, face down. It seems like my birthplace. The beginning of our village but changed. I see the eye, outlined, motionless, blue, without eyelashes. It goes away but I can see the shadow on the field. I do not see the eye any more. Everything is lost."

Post-hypnotic interview with the subject revealed the following:

After the initial induction the subject felt like his Self was opening up. He was moved and wanted to cry. Then he saw a huge yellow field that reminded him of the field where he used to play when he was a child. As soon as he entered the eye he went through a black space that also seemed light. He was eager to find what is beyond that point but was stopped by a huge brown door that was swimming in the air. He saw a man with a white beard and sparkling eyes who sent ocean waves to him and communicated with him telepathically. He understood that the door will not open. It is the "Door of Life" that will open after an eternity. He has to wait a long, long time. He cannot force it open.

These experiences were neither pleasant nor unpleasant ("these categories did not exist because it was something else"). The subject was reluctant to describe his experiences verbally because "these things are not possible to describe by words. By trying to describe, I am betraying them. Besides, I understood that I should not try to understand. These things are not subject to understanding."

After the session the subject felt like he had an emotional insight. As he confessed after two months in a follow-up interview, this experience made him review his system of existential values.

This researcher was so shocked and somewhat frightened by the unusual and unexpected nature of these responses that at some point during the experiment it was tempting to interrupt it. There was some kind of frightening solemn quality about all this not previously encountered in four years of practice with hypnosis. It penetrated through a system of conservative behavioral defenses and stirred something in this researcher's unconscious. Still reasonably skeptical, however, the research was continued.

Experimenting continued with the same stimulus word, as well as other images. Aside from the key transpersonal experiences reported above, a number of very provocative by-product effects also evolved. Subjects demonstrated an increased ability to manage their anxiety states, certain phobias, and existential growth and experienced emotional states similar to what are known as "peak and mystical experiences." These effects were all the more amazing considering their spontaneous character, in that no specific suggestions were presented to produce them in the experiments. Furthermore, content-analysis of symbols and images produced revealed certain stable and discernible cognitive emotional archetypal reaction patterns as described by C.G. Jung (Jung, 1959), and manifested in advance meditation practice (Goleman, 1984), clinical death experiences, and altered states of consciousness (Carr, 1993).

Thus, it became evident that granted certain conditions, specific symbolic stimuli words and images presented in deep hypnotic trance, definite unconscious patterns of reaction may emerge with subsequent spontaneous therapeutic effects. On the basis of this finding, the underlying assumption of Symbolic Experiential Training (SET) was defined: *with directed application of certain stimuli relevant to the collective unconscious it is possible to achieve therapeutic effects.* The next step of the research logically evolved from this basic assumption and consisted in the selection of appropriate collective unconscious symbols and images. This task was accomplished by:

- Developing criteria for the selection of collective unconscious material; and
- Reviewing and analyzing collective unconscious symbols/images as manifested in dreams, meditation practice, deep hypnotic trance, mythology, fairy-tales and critical and mystical experiences. The selected material was further tested in a series of pilot studies in actual SET practice.

Dimensions

SET is comprised of three hierarchically-arranged, relatively independent system subgoals or dimensions.

a. Basic Skills Dimension: This is the elementary or technical dimension of SET. It implies the development of a specific set of inter-related basic skills required to attain prerequisites of SET practice. In terms of the rationale used with SET patients and clients, this dimension provides "the key to open the door" to subsequent dimensions of SET. The subgoals relevant to this dimension involved: development of concentration and relaxation skills through autogenic exercises of heaviness, warmth, and breathing, as well as other imagery techniques, such as self-management of defenses and pathogenic states and self-administration of the acquired skills individual practices.

b. Personality Dimension: This is the intermediate dimension of SET. It involves gradual assimilation of personal unconscious or subconscious contents and is ultimately aimed at personality integration through harmonization of the conscious-unconscious continuum. The latter is accomplished by a structured set of self-examination, self-awareness and self-acceptance exercises, or "Trips," as well as by self-induced, self-monitored "Voyages into the Self." Accordingly, the subgoals of this dimension involve self-awareness and assimilation of the repressed, self-acceptance, personality growth and integration and independent SET practice skills development.

      c. Transpersonal Dimension: This is the advanced dimension of SET practice. It includes the following subgoals:

1. Awareness of the transpersonal and/or spiritual dimension of human existence and behavior inherent in the collective unconscious or higher forms of consciousness.
2. Actualization and utilization of this potential for self transcendence, spiritual or existential growth, and being-values motivation (Maslow, 1977).
3. Skills of effortless, fast self-administration of SET through a set of special, individualized symbol-image combinations.

Although hierarchically arranged so as to permit gradual progress from basic skills to transpersonal dimension, it goes without saying that these dimensions are closely inter-related as parts of a whole, continuous progress. In this respect, their differentiation is just a matter of theoretical convenience. In the actual practice of SET, the emergence of different subgoals varies both in terms of time and place in the overall structure.

Operational Aspects

      SET is a self-oriented system of intervention, i.e., it is based on the assumption that clients *can be taught* self-help and self-improvement skills. Unlike most of the hetero-oriented models of psychotherapy which heavily rely on the personality and professional skill of the therapist through the doctor-patient relationship, the self-oriented approach of SET implies greater freedom and utilization of internal healing resources inherent in the client. Accordingly, progress in SET suggests gradual autonomization of the client, starting with a modified individual reproduction of semi-directively induced states to fully independent choice of self-induction techniques, specific symbol-image combinations, and free-floating spontaneous expression. In fact, in advance stages of SET, the therapist's functions fade away fully, and are replaced by the client's individual, independent practice. Thus, as distinct from the hetero-oriented model of therapy, one of the principal goals of SET is to eliminate any evident or latent dependency from the therapist by progressive internalization of intervention techniques. The freedom and autonomy of the SET client also allows more room for the emergence of authentic, person-specific, spontaneous coping and self-regulation mechanisms.

Another operational principle of SET is based on what can be briefly defined as trust in the Inner World of Wisdom or Felt Sense (Gerdlin, 1978) that implies overcoming "the primitive fear of and aversion of everything that borders on the unconscious" (Jung, 1959), as well as "faith and confidence in a certain experience of an ominous nature and in the change of consciousness that ensues" (Jung, 1959). In other words, this is what in mindfulness meditation is called "choiceless awareness" and "self-accepting mindfulness" (Levine, 1989). In terms of SIT rationale, the principle of trust sounds as "Whatever happens is for the best. Whatever you think, feel, experience is for the best. The only thing you really have to do is do nothing. Just give yourself away to your own free-floating stream, let yourself go like a small boat to a huge, wide river."

Consistent with this rationale, no rigid or cut and dry operational structure has been drawn for SET to avoid unnecessary dogmatization. Instead, it relies on the individual experience and progress of each client, providing just the basic network principles for composing each consecutive stage and session. The latter suggests the extreme importance of the therapist or instructor factor. As a matter of fact, the SET instructor is required to have mastered at least those dimensions of the technique that he/she is going to teach. This is all the more indispensable because SET was not designed to be a directive technique of behavioral manipulation, but a process of mutual emotional sharing. This is sharing that implies natural interpersonal congruence of interacting subjects. Seen in terms of SET rationale, this is manifest as: "I am not going to lead you from the height of my 'Wisdom.' I will just be there with you." Likewise, a necessary condition of conducting SET sessions for the therapist/instructor is to simultaneously experience the states that need be induced or suggested. For this reason, no technical texts of SET sessions are ever provided, but merely the sequences of symbol/image units and combinations subject to induction.

Illustrative Results and Outcome Observations

It is certainly hard to draw a clear-cut demarcation line between different SET dimensions, as the process of gradual change and transformation includes all the layers of personality as a whole. Clearly then, a transformation emerging on one dimension simultaneously generates spontaneous changes on the others. Consequently, categorization of changes during SET practice suggests a well-known degree of theoretical relativity.

SET was successfully applied with a variety of patient and client populations for treatment and self-development purposes. It was also extensively used to relieve symptoms of PTSD in earthquake victim survivors from Armenia and Los Angeles.

On the level of Basic Skill Dimension, SET has proven effective in relieving symptoms of simple and social phobia, PTSD and adjustment disorders. Aside from its therapeutic significance, SET has also been found useful for pain control, enhancement of work potential, reduction of fatigability and general relaxation (Kalayjian, 1993). According to a self-report of a patient diagnosed with PTSD who completed the Basic Skills Dimension, "Sessions of SET awakened me, inspired, motivated, dissipated my disturbing thoughts and took me into a world where there is no earthquake, no fear, no orphans and no sad eyes."

The main effects of the Personality Dimension are associated with enhanced self-awareness, self-acceptance, field independence, facilitation of creative potential and improved self-management and coping skills. In this respect the following extract from an interview with a highly introverted male client who was experiencing severe anxiety and existential problems might be illustrative. "You know, it seemed like my Self standing there presented with different riddles that I had to solve. At some point I saw a man that was burning and radiating light. When I asked myself how does that "Sun-Man" preserve himself when he is burning all the time, he said that the energy and the light are being reciprocated. Because of that cycle he stays alive. The same is true for life. You must get back the energy you transmit, not in an egotistical sense, but by creating something, or, for example, looking at nature."

The most challenging and intriguing effects of SET, however, are associated with the Transpersonal Dimension. Changes like mindfulness or expansion of awareness, enhancement, cognitive vs. perceptual content discrimination, "anatta" or "non-self" consciousness widely known in meditation theory, emerge abundantly. Furthermore, in-depth actualization of inherent creative potential, peak and mystical experiences with ensuing personality transformations, self-transcendence and existential growth are observed to occur. SET subjects who have reached this stage also develop an ability to self induce spontaneously desired SET states without external assistance. The following poem written by one of the SET clients would best describe the richness and authenticity of this dimension:

"Remaining the Same,
Being the Same,
I grow,
I continue."

Prospects for Development

The process of SET development is still in progress. It is expected to be in progress as long as it is practiced by any particular client or therapist because SET's growth potential lies in its very structure and logistics. Accordingly, none of the SET aspects described above are considered to be a priority or predetermined. Much work yet needs to be done in the area of symbol/image selection, SET dimensions, principles, and, of course, in improving the theoretical framework of interpretation.

The creative nature of SET, coupled with the universality of its proposed psychological mechanisms, would also make it a potent cross-cultural tool of therapeutic intervention. One might consider, in this respect, the possibility of cross-cultural controlled research.

In summary, then, SET is still in the process of developing and enduring. It awaits scrupulous researchers, inventive proponents, and, most importantly, critical opponents.

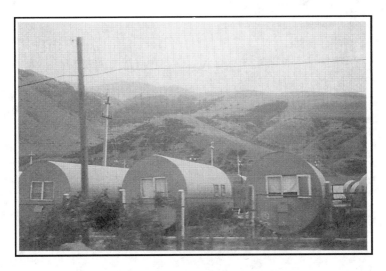

Nine months hence: Still housed in temporary shelters
survivors of Leninakan brace for the
harsh Armenian winter ahead
August, 1989

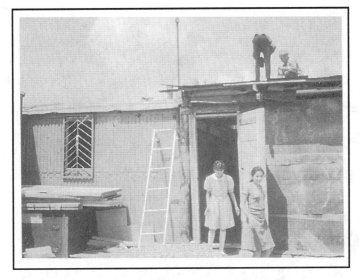

Fifteen months hence: Survivors of the 1988 Armenian quake
emerge from their make shift shelters
having endured their first post-quake
winter.
April, 1990
Photographs by: Dr. Anie Sanentz Kalayjian

135

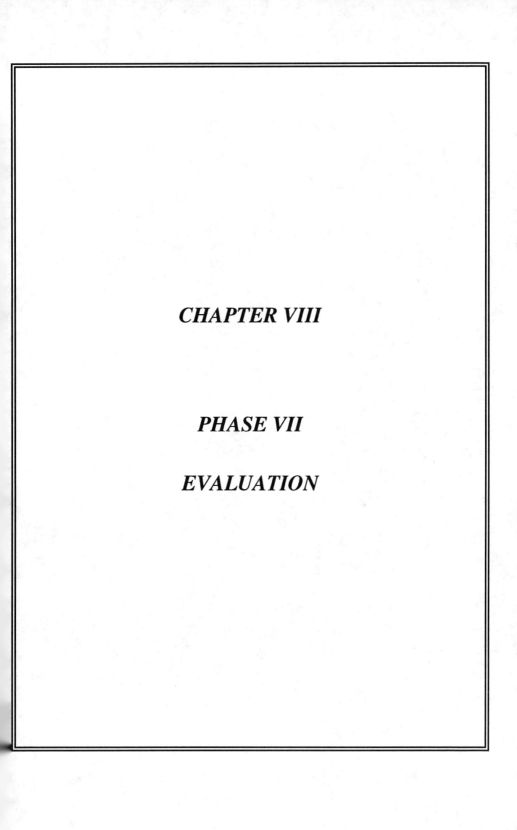

CHAPTER VIII

PHASE VII

EVALUATION

CHAPTER VIII

Some people regard themselves as perfect,
but only because they demand little of themselves.

Herman Hesse

PHASE VII

EVALUATION

Evaluation is the seventh phase of MHOP. This phase will directly follow the implementation of action. During this phase the author determined the progress and effectiveness of the care provided. MHOP is cyclic; after the evaluation it leads to remodification, which in turn will lead back to the beginning of the program meaning assessment.

In this phase the mental health professional focuses on three measures:
1. Changes experienced by the survivors;
2. Changes reported by significant others;
3. The quality of the care provided as reported by the caregivers.

Expert mental health professionals are the most appropriate to conduct the evaluation. Depending on the size of the outreach program, evaluation can take one week, to one month; the faster the better, since the information from the evaluation phase is utilized in the next, remodification phase.

Short Term

Approximately six months into the short-term implementation phase it was necessary to evaluate the Mental Health Outreach Program. The author traveled to Armenia to conduct an on-site evaluation six months and then again one year after the disaster. Six months and then one year follow-up research studies were also conducted after Hurricane Andrew. The rationale for this evaluation is as follows:
1. Human behavior and therapeutic care is a dynamic process. Many events may cause a change or alteration in the assessment, diagnosis or plans made previously.
2. Evaluation is a process examining the need and worth of the plan.

3. Evaluation determines the degree to which the plan had been effective and useful.

In the evaluation phase, communication with several layers of the community is necessary to investigate the effectiveness of the plan. The following people need be involved:

1. Clients, families and their significant others.
2. Providers of the therapeutic care, i.e., teachers, therapists, physicians
3. Community leaders, as well as leaders of voluntary organizations
4. Government officials, armed forces and rescue workers.

Armenia
Six month follow-up

A six month follow-up evaluation conducted by this author in Armenia revealed that those survivors (n = 180) who received care by the MHOP's professional teams were:

1. Coping more effectively (78%), based on one-to-one interviews and the survivors' own anecdotal reports.
2. Less depressed (50%), based on the interview process and the survivors' own observations.
3. Scored lower on the PTSD Reaction Index Scale (80%). (Kalayjian, 1994)

In comparison, those survivors who did not receive care from the MHOP's professional teams expressed feelings of hopelessness, helplessness, anger, despair and apathy. These same survivors, immediately after the quake, were working together cohesively, struggling to survive, helping one another and hoping that, with the coming of spring, they would spring back to a more stable life. Instead, they had nothing but tanks, tents and makeshift sheds for basic shelter, air polluted with dust due to the rubble, no running water in many places for 15 hours a day, and no electricity for several hours a day. Only about 50% of the survivors had homes, 30% were in shelters and the remaining 20% had relocated to other parts of what was then the Soviet Union or to the United States.

Those who did not benefit from the MHOP or did not receive any psychological support continued exhibiting signs of moderate to severe levels of PTSD. The incidence of suicide, homicide, aggressive outbursts, substance abuse, and spousal and child abuse had increased. Less than 15% of the projected construction had been completed in the quake zone. Almost all aid from around the world subsided, and the Azeri blockade continued.

The following are some of the contributing factors as to why some survivors did not participate in the Mental Health Outreach Program:

1. The geographic distance of survivors from the outreach centers.
2. The survivor/mental health professional ratio.
3. The new modality, that of a "talking cure," a concept foreign to the survivors.
4. The priority for those survivors was obtaining food, shelter and clean air to breath.
5. Resistance to treatment and toward authority figures.
6. Resistance to foreigners.

The author then recommended the following interventions:

- Collaborate with and motivate American philanthropic organizations which have enormous resources at their disposal to expedite the reconstruction process. The author began a campaign to inform the public by submitting articles to newspapers and appearing on local radio and television shows to raise the motivation of Americans and Armenian-Americans to continue their financial support of Armenia.
- Continue on-site clinical interventions using the MHOP professional teams for longer stays. The longer time would allow for follow-up and long-term treatments.
- Engage in on-site education and training of teachers, psychologists, psychiatrists and other health professionals, as well as invite them to the United States. The purpose of this emphasis is to reach a larger number of survivors and to empower Armenia's professionals by providing them with the necessary instruments, knowledge and expertise in PTSD to help themselves and their communities.
- Develop community mental health clinics in the affected cities of Leninakan, Kirovakan and Spitak in order to provide easy access to care for the community.
- Collaborate with the mental health professionals in Armenia and Moscow to conduct joint research studies.
- Provide training and orientation for those professionals providing field relief work in Armenia and upon their return, provide them with support groups and debriefing sessions.

Florida
Six month follow-up

A six month follow-up study in Florida revealed that many communities were still in chaos. People were still "walking wounded," suffering emotionally from post-hurricane trauma. The author conducted research to indicate the level of PTSD. The Reaction Index Scale was the instrument utilized once again for its brevity and clarity to measure the level of PTSD and additional questions were asked in order to elicit what changes in survivors' personal and social lives had occurred.

The study sample consisted of 127 individuals who had survived Hurricane Andrew. Respondents were selected unintentionally from several shelters in Southern Florida, as well as South Miami Hospital at Homestead.

Survivors described experiencing a multitude of coping difficulties. Although three months post-hurricane the survivors reported going through normal reactions to a massive trauma such as grieving for their losses, struggling to address the daily obstacles, helping one another, and receiving help from others, six months later they were overwhelmed by feelings of uncertainty and despair. Some began to rely on substances to alleviate or numb their pain and suffering, saying to themselves, "There is no use, I might as well get drunk." Others became short-tempered and irritable and began physically and verbally abusing each other. Domestic violence increased, as did spousal and child abuse. Responses such as, "She irritates me so much, I can't take it anymore," were common for situations of child abuse. Those who did not have a spouse or children reported abusing their pet dogs and cats. However, those survivors who had positive meaning associated with the disaster, about 22% of those interviewed, coped in a more healthy manner.

Analysis of variance revealed strong correlation's between PTSD and education, with significance at $<.001$; PTSD and severity of damage to home, significance at $<.001$; education and helplessness, significance at $.005$; employment and helplessness, significance at $.003$; with PTSD and meaning significance at $.003$.

Long Term

Over the year following the earthquake in Armenia, dozens of mental health professionals volunteered and went to Armenia to continue on-site clinical interventions. They provided supportive interventions to over 10,000 survivors in the quake zone. Mobile clinics were established in the villages and towns. Permanent outpatient clinics were founded in Leninakan, Kirovakan and Spitak. Many of the author's recommendations were carried out. However, the housing project progressed very slowly; Armenia had other priorities to address. Among them were:

1. The border war with Azerbaijan
2. The Azeri blockade; that was stopping 80% of the goods from entering Armenia;
3. Housing the over 300,000 Armenian refugees who fled Azerbaijan; and
4. The constant changes in leadership, due to the fight for democracy.

Armenia
One year follow-up

The author returned to Armenia in April 1991 to evaluate the MHOP and gather more data for the ongoing research. The outpatient clinics in Leninakan (managed by Earthquake Relief Fund for Armenia (ERFA)) and Kirovakan (managed by SOS Armenia) were in place. Both clinical care and training were taking place. Two MHOP team members were staying in Armenia for one year each, to supervise, train and conduct clinical work. About 40% of the survivors who visited the clinic had severe PTSD and 15% suffered from major depressive disorders. According to Vasken Manoukian (Kalayjian, 1991d), the then Prime Minister of Armenia, only 19% of the housing had been completed, leaving thousands of Armenian refugees in need of housing. About 90% of the refugees interviewed by this author had severe levels of PTSD. They had escaped the beating, rapes and torture by the Azerbaijanis.

Florida
One Year Follow-Up

One year after Hurricane Andrew was an especially stressful time for the Floridians. Haunting memories of Hurricane Andrew and its impact and the fear of yet another hurricane tormented many residents of South Dade County, where post-hurricane stress was still as apparent as the gnarled street signs and empty shopping malls. Many of the Andrew survivors found themselves drinking heavily, fighting with family members or co-workers, and panicking over a thunderstorm. Some still had nightmares, woke up screaming at night, could not concentrate, and could not engage in their pre-hurricane hobbies.

Spousal and child abuse increased in Dade County and the divorce rate rose by a reported 30%. This author's one year follow-up interview findings of close to one hundred survivors, were consistent with the above findings. The number of domestic violence suits filed in 1992 in Dade Circuit Court reached 4,586, about double the number from the previous year. One survivor said, "My husband drinks more and more now after the hurricane, and when he drinks he is violent toward me."

The schools in Dade County had experienced a tremendous increase in the frequency of suicide attempts. According to Joseph Jackson, supervisor of psychological services for the Dade County schools, there were 19 suicide attempts among young children in less than one year after Andrew, as compared to two attempts a year before the hurricane. Some very small children had regressed in their toilet training and verbal skills. Some remained fearful to sleep alone, afraid of loud noises and all storms.

The media was focused heavily on two tropical depressions, numbers 5 and 6, which were in the Atlantic Ocean, and heading west. Of course, reporters added a few days later that neither one of them was an immediate threat to Florida. Tropical Storm Cindy, which churned through the Caribbean, was another threat. FEMA checked the inventory of relief supplies such as refrigerated trucks, generators, pumps and medical equipment, as well as the opening of telephone lines to the state's emergency response team in Tallahassee. In the end, the storm veered south and eventually died. This was an enormous improvement for FEMA, after a botched response post-hurricane Andrew.

According to authorities one year after Hurricane Andrew, nearly 12,000 people still had no place to live. Others whose homes were destroyed had moved into mobile homes provided by FEMA, even though mobile homes were 21 times more likely to be destroyed by hurricanes than regular houses. The Cutler Ridge area was 50% rebuilt, except for the shopping mall. Miami hotels, which served as homes for many displaced residents, did well. Overall, the tourism industry revived rather rapidly in Dade County.

The survivors were additionally traumatized by the practices of insurance companies, federal agencies, looters, robbers and construction workers. Experts call this "secondary traumatization." The American Psychological Association had issued a warning to disaster victims that the anniversary dates of disasters can reactivate thoughts and feelings from the actual event and that survivors may experience a resurgence of symptoms such as anxiety, depression, helplessness, frustration and loss of control.

Homestead Air Force Base, once home to 8,000 active military and civilian workers, had only about 200 people working there, as officials planned its rebirth as a military reserve post and general aviation center. The tent cities and more than 29,000 troops and reserve units deployed at the peak of the recovery were gone, along with the long lines for water, food, mail and gas. Out of the 47,000 houses and apartments destroyed in Dade County, only 15,000 had been repaired. Of the dislocated 101,000 residents, only two thirds had returned. Officials estimate it will take until the turn of the century for the population to return to pre-Andrew levels.

As for employment, of the 60,000 jobs lost in Dade County following the hurricane, only one third had returned. But, fortunately, country-wide employment had actually increased by 4.5% since Andrew, and sales tax proceeds have soared due to the rebuilding efforts. 7,236 claims for disaster unemployment assistance were submitted and $12.4 million was disbursed.

Although the last hurricane of Andrew's size was Donna in 1960, this first anniversary had left Floridians especially uneasy, anxious and even paranoid. FEMA reported taking steps to ease the fears and uncertainty by educating and preparing the residents. A statewide campaign on hurricane preparedness was launched at this time.

Floridians and FEMA have developed a better understanding since Andrew, assuring that following a natural disaster, joint damage assessment teams would be on the ground within ten hours. FEMA has since learned to work very closely with state disaster agencies and has found quicker means by which to provide aid to disaster victims. FEMA is expected to stay in Southern Florida for at least 2 or 3 years. They have spent over $2.1 billion on the recovery from Hurricane Andrew, with about $3 billion allocated. Another $5 billion will be spent by other federal agencies on economic development, agriculture and social services. One year after the hurricane, FEMA reported that more than 90% of the nearly 47,000 requests for housing assistance had been settled.

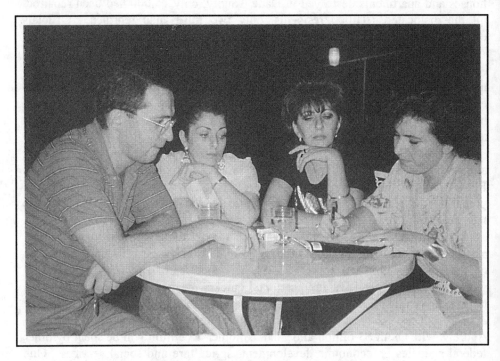

One year hence: Dr. Anie Sanentz Kalayjian and mental health professionals from
Armenia huddle to assess the progress of the MHOP,
with an eye towards remodification.
Yerevan, Armenia
1989

Photograph by: Dr. Sarisarkis Zakarian

CHAPTER IX

PHASE VIII

REMODIFICATION

CHAPTER IX

Whatever authority I may have,
Rests solely on knowing how
little I know.

Socrates

PHASE VIII

REMODIFICATION

Remodification is the last phase of MHOP. It directly follows the evaluation phase. This is a process of tailoring the plan especially to fit the needs of individual survivors and the survivor community. In this phase it is important to take the following steps:

1. Identify areas of deficit
2. Prioritize the problem list
3. Identify new interventions
4. Implement
5. Reevaluate
6. Remodify

In Armenia:

According to this author's observations and evaluations, there is the need for at least a twenty-year continued on-site clinical intervention program with three groups:

1. The earthquake survivors;
2. The refugees from Azerbaijan; and,
3. The former government's Communist Party leaders who were expressing feelings of shame, doubt, defeat, resentment, uncertainty due to the collapse of the Soviet Union.

In Armenia, when addressing the educational arena, it is recommended that a twenty-year plan be established for schools in clinical psychology, social work and nursing, as well as training programs in interpersonal and behavioral modalities. For example, the Armenian General Benevolent Union and the University of California have founded the American University of Armenia. It opened its doors in the Fall of 1991, offering M.A. degrees in business, industrial engineering and earthquake engineering. Future programs could be in the fields of clinical psychology with specialty programs in social work, counseling and psychiatric nursing.

In Florida and California, fortunately, there was no need for the development of new programs or schools as there were ample educational institutions, as well as training programs in disaster management. In the United States, increased focus needs to be placed on research programs with follow-up research studies to contribute to the understanding of disaster impact and disaster response. Due to the technological and scientific advancement in both Florida and California, remodification from outside was not essential. Mental health professionals within the surviving communities took charge and outside interventions were not needed.

In California:

Although much attention was placed on the earthquake zone immediately after the event, more work was needed, especially when the broadcasters stopped showing the devastating scenes and the newspapers stopped printing articles about the quake.

Months after the earthquake of January 17, 1994, staff nurses at Santa Monica Hospital spoke at a press conference hosted by California Assemblyman Burt Margolin (D-Los Angeles), regarding legislation calling for increased safety standards for all hospitals in California. The Hospital Seismic Safety Act holds hospitals to stricter standards than other buildings, but applies only to hospitals built after 1973. Although health care facilities and hospitals are expected to be less vulnerable and more prepared to deal with emergency situations, during the last two decades more than one hundred hospitals in the Americas have reported severe disruptions, or total collapse, as a result of earthquakes. During the San Fernando, California, earthquake of February 9, 1971, four hospitals were damaged so severely that they were no longer operational. In addition, the majority of deaths caused by that earthquake occurred in two of the collapsed hospitals. Therefore, it is imperative to consider increased safety standards for all hospitals; perhaps by applying the Hospital Seismic Safety Act to all hospitals regardless of their age.

Immediately after the quake, basic needs for food, shelter, and clean air had been addressed. In mid-March, about two months after the quake, the longer-term needs of the survivors had been addressed, such as permanent housing, relocation, repairs and crisis intervention. This period is generally expected to last at least one year post-quake.

Many organizations are supporting employees and their families post-disaster. For example, the California Nurses Association contributed to the relief efforts by establishing an Earthquake Relief Fund within the California Nurses Foundation. This fund provided monetary assistance to nurses, nursing students and vulnerable and disadvantaged populations not served by other relief efforts.

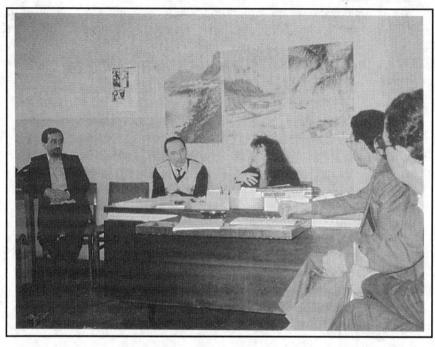

Two years hence: Dr. Anie Sanentz Kalayjian shares her research findings with
leading scientists.
Yerevan, Armenia
1990

Photograph by: Dr. Sarkisarkis Zakarian

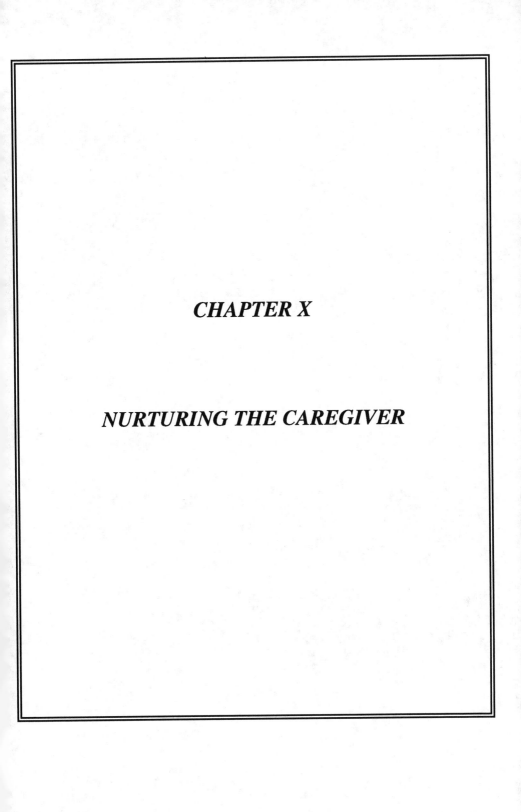

CHAPTER X

NURTURING THE CAREGIVER

CHAPTER X

He who has a why to live
Can bear with almost any how.

Frederich Nietzsche

NURTURING THE CAREGIVER

EDUCATION AND TRAINING

One of the essential methods in providing support to mental health professionals and survivors regarding disasters is providing education and information. Three of this author's research study findings revealed that survivors valued information as an important support to cope with the natural disaster response. Sharing information could occur on several levels, such as through formal and informal education, training, conferences, workshops and networking.

Information sharing and dissemination must be an integral part of disaster management. Although this aspect of disaster has been addressed in most disaster-prone areas of the United States, more emphasis should be placed on vulnerable groups, such as refugees, legal and illegal aliens, children, the elderly and tourists. Training materials must be in the language of the community and the reading level must be congruent to those levels reflected in the community.

In the United States, especially during the last decade, many more private and community organizations have developed and sponsored community outreach projects, distributed handouts and educational materials and provided training opportunities.

The following are some examples of organizations providing disaster training programs, workshops and courses in their communities:

1. *The American Institute of Architects.*
2. *The Building Seismic Safety Council.*
3. *The Applied Technology Council.*
4. *The Earthquake Engineering Research Institute.*
5. *The National Information Service for Earthquake Engineering at the University of California at Berkeley and California Institute of Technology.*

6. *The Information Services of the National Center for Earthquake Engineering Research.*
7. *The American Red Cross.*
8. *United Nations Department of Humanitarian Affairs.*
9. *Pan American Health Organization, regional office of World Health Organization (WHO).*

Several states have formed or are in the process of forming Seismic Advisory Boards and Seismic Safety Councils. The purpose of these committees is to promote mitigation measures, distribute disaster specific maps, brochures, and handouts, as well as design earthquake safety programs, drills and annual awareness campaigns in schools, hospitals and community centers. The State of Utah, for example, has developed a disaster mitigation handbook which addresses all natural hazards in Utah, including earthquakes, flash floods and wildfires. The State of California has developed many handouts in regard to earthquakes. It is recommended that other states developed similar age-appropriate handbooks addressing the hazard information needs of their communities. Professional associations, among them the American Psychiatric Association and Psychological Association, as well as the International Society for Traumatic Stress Studies, have also printed materials for disaster education (see Chapter XI).

Annual conferences and workshops are also used to add to the formal training and preparation, to update the technological information and to share recent research findings. The following recent conferences in the United states and abroad are worthy of mention:

- The Annual National Hurricane Conference.
- The United States Pacific Insular States Earthquake and Hurricane Conference (by the Pacific Region Emergency Management Caucus).
- The National Dam Safety Program.
- The Forest Services (The US National Report, 1994).
- World Conference on Natural Disaster, Japan, 1994.
- United Nations, Department of Humanitarian Affairs, Moscow, 1991 and Frunze 1990.
- International Society for Traumatic Stress Studies: World, national and regional conferences.
- American Orthopsychiatric Association, National Conferences.
- American Psychiatric Association Annual Conferences.
- American Psychological Association Annual Conferences.

Due to the nature of the demands made upon the caregiver who volunteers in disaster situations, it is essential to ensure, as much as possible, that this outreach is a meaningful experience. The focus of this chapter is on educating, preparing, nurturing and supporting the caregiver. What follows is a preparatory process from inception to closure.

The work of Braak deals with formal training opportunities for the caregiver. She provides the names of leading training programs throughout the country and details characteristic traits of trauma workers.

In an adaptation of the 12 steps of recovery of Alcoholics Anonymous (AA), Brende has developed a program of recovery for victims of disaster. He also articulates the four elements of debriefing, which is an essential part of the relief process.

In an attempt to offer support to caregivers who work with survivors, Danieli has provided a group therapy model for processing counter transferencial issues. Danieli's writing, although based on her work with therapists working on Nazi Holocaust survivors, is equally relevant to therapists working with more acute or recent trauma survivors.

In the next section, on fostering resiliency in disaster responders, Dunnings challenges the crisis intervention theory as a framework. Based on her experience, not all effects of trauma are negative. She prefers the wellness model with its focus on hardiness and resiliency, since some long-term effects of the trauma experience are life enhancing instead of life depleting.

The final offering by Karakashian and Mercer is a pilot study of survivors who also served as counselors. After the 1988 earthquake in Armenia, Karakashian offered seven didactic classes on theory and treatment of trauma to the counselors. The preliminary findings indicate a reduction in depression and PTSD symptoms. Further research with a larger sample was recommended by the authors.

With almost a decade of experience as both caregiver and trauma worker, the author has generated guidelines for preparing trauma workers.

Guidelines for Preparing Trauma Volunteers

The Selection Process:

Before the on-site assessment, the author placed a news release in various relevant newspapers in the United States, Canada and the Middle East, seeking volunteer mental health professionals fluent in the Armenian language to go to Armenia to assist. Due to the urgent nature of the assignment, the volunteers were instructed to respond immediately. Within fifteen days, the author had received approximately fifty completed applications. An application eliciting the availability of the volunteers, the length of time able to designate for this outreach, amount of time needed prior to departure, theoretical and clinical focus, type of degree and licensure, in addition to other demographic information was distributed (see Appendix H).

Based on the three factors listed above, a subgroup was selected (Group 1A). Those candidates for the on-site outreach who were experts in disaster management were called for an interview. Those candidates who were expert but who were not fluent in the Armenian language were placed in Group II.

I. *General Announcement*:

1. Place a news release in all relevant papers, as well as on air, requesting volunteers.
2. Place a volunteer application form in all relevant papers.
3. Mail volunteer application to mental health professions, using directories of professional organization (see Appendix H).

II. *The Interview*:

Due to the wide geographical distribution and time constraints, most of the interviews were conducted on the telephone. The interviews ranged from one hour to four hours, within an average of two hours. The author contacted applicants in Group 1A within 48-72 hours after the receipt of the applications. The interview had five objectives. The objectives of the interview were:

1. To elicit the motivation of the volunteer and to rule out self-aggrandizing motives (Why would you like to volunteer at this time?).
2. To elicit previous positive resolution of traumatic experience (What are your related experiences in trauma? How did you resolve those experiences?).
3. To elicit past experience in psychotherapy/supervision and willingness to see assistance as needed (How prepared are you emotionally and psychologically? What would you do if you were unable to deal with the experience?).
4. To elicit present social/family interpersonal support (Where are you developmentally? Who is there for you when you need support?).
5. To elicit the volunteer's expectations of this experience.

Based on the above five objectives, the following profile was developed describing necessary personal experiences of the volunteer.

151

A. Related Personal Experiences:

1. Previous experience in a similar (disaster) situation (as survivor or caregiver).
2. Previous experiences in disaster outreach.
3. Travel and/or work in foreign countries.
4. Previous positive resolution of a traumatic experience.
5. Past history of clinical supervision/psychotherapy, group therapy.
6. Willingness to seek clinical supervision/psychotherapy as needed.

B. Inclusion Criteria:

The literature on the characteristics of effective mental health professionals (Schaffer, 1982; Rogers, 1957; and Strupp, Hadley & Gomes-Schwartz, 1977), and experiences with Armenia, Florida and California, assisted this author in outlining a set of attributes and life experiences of potentially effective mental health caregivers. In addition to degree, licensure and experience, the following attributes were found essential (not listed in order of importance):

1. Assertive
2. Humorous
3. Able to deal with the unknown and the uncertain
4. Good listener
5. Non judgmental, open to accept differences
6. High energy with a positive attitude
7. Supportive and generous with compliments
8. Problem solver, with alternate plans in place
9. Caring and compassionate
10. Nurturing to self and others
11. Organized in thinking and action
12. Self-motivated and able to motivate others easily
13. Collaborative and cooperative
14. Physically fit and mentally stable

Given the time pressure, the interview may be a limited vehicle to assess all the characteristics outlined above. During the course of the author's experience working with over fifty mental health volunteers from Armenia, Southern Florida and Southern California, the need for exclusion criteria became apparent.

C. Exclusion Criteria:

1. Fulfilling grandiose personal needs
2. Proselytism: Religious and/or political
3. Pursuing business investments, i.e., export/import, real estate
4. Pursuing spousal/marital relationships
5. Having health complications: psychiatric and/or physical illnesses or disabilities requiring continuous observation
6. Engaging in scholarly pursuits without collaboration with the team

The initial assessment of the volunteer was the most difficult step for this author, since the majority of the interviews were on the telephone. Due to the limited number of professional mental health caregivers who were fluent in Armenian, the author had to reach out to volunteers in Canada, Europe and distant parts of the United States. The process was financially draining, since the author's telephone bills ranged from $200-350 US dollars per month.

Team work is highly recommended, within an established organization such as CARE, FEMA, the Red Cross, the United Nations or the World Health Organization.

III. Preparing the Caregiver

The orientation phase: Group 1A
Materials to distribute during the orientation:

1. Research studies related to the disaster
2. Initial assessment report conducted by the administrators
3. Names of contact persons at the disaster site
4. Names of contact persons for leisure activities at the disaster site
5. Personal accounts and vignettes
6. Stationeries, supplies and other necessities
7. Emergency chain of command

An orientation began providing research articles related to the disaster at hand. This served as a vehicle for empowerment. Similarities and differences in responses to the disaster were discussed. For example, according to other research on earthquake trauma, survivors had not expressed feelings of anger, unlike earthquake survivors in Armenia, the majority of whom did express anger.

Other handouts and pamphlets related to the disaster at hand were not only helpful to the caregivers, but helpful to the survivors who were also empowered by this information. Additionally, the initial assessment report was used as a guide, in that it detailed the impact of the disaster at hand. For example, the initial assessment report regarding the earthquake in Armenia was based on an evaluation of 213 adults, 126 adolescents and 122 children from Spitak, Leninakan (now Gumri), and Kirovakan (see Chapter IV).

Names of contact persons facilitate the on -site experience of the caregiver. This is especially important in a foreign country, where one does not know whom to trust, who has the resources and who has the positional power. The contacts were persons whom the author had met, worked with, presented the Mental Health Outreach Plan to, and who had agreed to collaborate. These contacts were people with resources, and positional power and most were mental health professionals.

Contact persons for leisure activity were also essential. The author realized the importance of leisure and relaxation after working 12-16 hour days in a chaotic, highly stressful disaster environment. Caregivers need therapeutic outlets, at least one day a week. Since every community has its beautiful parks, mountains, lakes or rivers, the local residents are best suited to help the caregiver to move out of the disaster environment, and unwind by experiencing aesthetic beauty and breathing clean, fresh air. These natives provided the caregivers with a therapeutic outlet and were helped themselves by feeling important and special, since they had the privilege of hosting the caregivers and the opportunity to reciprocate the hosting.

The author's personal experience made the orientation especially real. One question that was asked by almost all caregivers: How did the survivors respond to you? Was there any resistance? No research study can help answered this question better than personal experience. Almost always, survivors were very receptive, open and expressive. The only resistance was from the local government bureaucrats in all three areas (Armenia, Southern Florida and Southern California).

The most effective way to deal with resistance is to expect it, work with it, instead of fighting against it. Making leaders feel comfortable, secure and trusting is essential. One way to make them feel secure is to identify their leadership strengths and acknowledging them. Another effective approach is to focus on mutual goals and work toward their accomplishment.

Caregivers were instructed to take with them items such as paper pads, drawing paper, pencils, pens, markers, crayons, work books, pamphlets, the *Physician's Desk Reference* (PDR), as well as any other items they felt were helpful. These items facilitated the working experience by providing the necessary equipment to the caregivers. Crayons and markers attracted the children and adolescents; pamphlets helped the adults as well as educators and parents; PDR's empowered the professionals to understand the actions and side effects of American medications.

Finally, caregivers learned how to contact their families in case of emergency. Since disasters usually cause varying degrees of infrastructure damage, it is essential to have an emergency communication plan in place.

Volunteer caregivers were asked to keep a journal, to log their own feelings and experiences, dreams and anecdotal cases. This practice not only assisted the caregiver in the therapeutic process, but also served as an avenue for debriefing.

Volunteer caregivers were also asked to write a report at the end of their rotation to be used as a means of orientation for the next team, and as an update for the MHOP administrators.

Caregivers' reports included the following information:

- Census
- Demographics
- Hours logged in per day
- Clinical impressions and interventions
- Follow-up
- Changes in contact persons/leadership
- Recommendations for the next team
- Recommendations for the administrators

Applicants in group II were utilized in the following way:

- As resources for trauma literature
- As support for the administrators of the program
- As debriefers for the volunteers and administrators
- As assistants in the research process
- As assistants in the publication and dissemination of information

IV. Return of the Caregiver

A. Debriefing and support:

Upon the return of each group of volunteer caregivers, a debriefing and supportive session was conducted. When geographically feasible, the entire team was included; when not feasible, individual sessions were conducted either face-to-face or on the telephone. Each volunteer received at least one mandatory hour-long session. Follow-up sessions were provided as needed.

These sessions included time for emotional catharsis, support, providing further information and references regarding countertransferencial issues and restoration. Those volunteers who expressed willingness to return to the disaster site for another rotation were give further literature regarding treatment modalities for survivors needing follow-up treatments.

B. Celebration:

Upon the return of the caregiver it is essential to provide a public forum for acknowledgment and reward. Therefore, organized community presentations were held disseminating the work that the MHOP and the specific volunteers provided. Announcements were placed in local newspapers and on the radio regarding the nature and purpose of celebratory activity. Volunteers were often asked to present their experiences to the audience in ways most comfortable to them, such as videos, slides, photographs, children's drawings and lectures. Participants were encouraged to engage in a dialogue with the volunteers. New volunteers were generated in this process. At the end of the dialogue, a social hour followed with food and refreshments.

Frequently, communities acknowledged their own volunteers with plaques, awards, citations and gifts. Often volunteers were interviewed by journalists from a variety of newspapers, radio and television stations. Acknowledging and celebrating the work of volunteers is an essential final step within the process of volunteering. As the information was disseminated and celebrations continued, community empathy manifested itself in calls, donations and contributions.

C. Follow-up:

Three volunteers impressed this author with their resourcefulness by returning to Armenia for extended periods of time through Fulbright Fellowships. This provided the author a cadre of experienced and available volunteers to serve as disaster team leaders for future catastrophes. With the combination of research and extensive field experience, future relief will come expeditiously, effectively within the limitations of the political climate.

One must not hold one's self so divine
as to be unwilling occasionally
to make improvements in one's creations.

Ludwig van Beethoven

Training and Accreditation

Joyce Braak, MD

Catastrophe has always had an intense impact on human beings. Such dramatic events have historically been the raw material of journalists, historians, authors, poets, visual and performing artists and philosophers. These professionals have labored to describe, define, report and record, ponder, and interpret the catastrophe itself, and its devastation.

The awesome forces of nature, by contrast, underscore the relative fragility of human beings, but average persons in their daily routines are rarely conscious of this unwelcome reality. Even use of the term "Act of God" implies a power beyond that of humankind. For these and other reasons, the general public is, and probably has always been, fascinated by natural disasters, providing that this fascinated public is at a safe distance from the disaster.

Whenever a disaster occurs there are survivors. The survivors are people injured physically, emotionally or both, and require the attention and aid of others. What they require are people trained to respond to the crisis, to their needs, to their unique and specific situation. In addition to the self-evident medical and physical needs, survivors are simultaneously at risk of developing Post-traumatic Stress Disorder (PTSD) and consequent losses of functional capabilities. It has been reported that in the aftermath of a devastating disaster 50 to 80 percent of the survivors may suffer PTSD and its disabling symptoms. Effective response by trained providers can reduce this risk, and diminish severity of PTSD symptoms and future disability. The value of trained professionals available to respond to such crises seems reasonable and obvious.

So the question is, who are these trained crisis responders, and how are they trained? The answer must begin with a brief excursion into history.

Recognition of Post-traumatic Stress Disorder and the need for training and research in this special area has a short history relative to that of the traditional professions and their established formal education. Jacob DaCosta published a paper, "On Irritable Heart," describing a syndrome commonly called soldier's heart that was observed in Civil War soldiers; this syndrome was periodically noted as a malady of combat survivors. After research and attention to the sufferings of Vietnam Veterans and those of civilian trauma survivors, the diagnostic category Post-traumatic Stress Disorder (PTSD) was published in the *Diagnostic and Statistical Manual III* (APA, 1980).

Since that time, interest and research in this area has grown rapidly and robustly among individuals from multiple disciplines. This area, trauma and its survivors, is not the exclusive province of any one profession but rather a common interest of many. Pioneers eager to share their new knowledge with others, founded the Society for Traumatic Stress Studies (STSS), which matured to become the International Society for Traumatic Stress Studies (ISTSS). Even prior to that period, advocacy for crime victims was growing due to the efforts and energies of similar pioneers proceeding from a different perspective. The resultant organization is the National Organization for Victim Assistance (NOVA), a private, non-profit organization whose activities are guided by specific goals and purposes. More recently, the International Association of Trauma Counselors (IATC), was formed to meet the needs of its clinician members. The Red Cross, of course, has long been recognized for its efforts to meet the needs of civilian and military survivors in crisis situations and has also increased its focus to include the mental health needs of disaster survivors. Each of these organizations has paid attention to the need for focused and appropriate training for those who respond to the needs of traumatized people (see Appendix A and B).

Traditionally, the care of the injured individual is entrusted to those who have satisfactorily completed a defined formal education in their chosen profession. This traditional training, long-established, is based on certain assumptions about the circumstances in which help is sought and services are delivered. This formal professional education has also incorporated certain assumptions about the injured, disabled help-seeker, and the power or control balance in the treatment situation.

Natural disasters, by definition, cause a profound disruption of the physical environment. Normal individuals who did exist in a state of equilibrium become survivors. In the immediate aftermath, survivors may be so overwhelmed and shocked by the sense of powerlessness they feel, that they may not seek help. The assumptions of setting, pathology, and power or control balance on which traditionally circumscribed professional education's are founded may be equally shattered and disrupted. Generally, traditional education does not suffice to meet the needs of the survivors when a disaster has proven that the world we inhabit can alter abruptly, proving itself profoundly uncertain. In a disaster even the infrastructure of a community, those means taken for granted in customary professional practices can cease to exist. On-site, where the survivors are located, even drinking water can be scarce and precious. And, in a natural disaster, the local trained professionals also become survivors, imposed role that takes precedence over all else.

Clearly, specialized training for these crises is required, but this is a new field of knowledge. Professional education and licensure do not automatically qualify an individual to respond appropriately to a disaster. There is an enormous need for flexibility in the responder. Recently, IATC president, Tom Williams, an experienced crisis responder, compiled a list of the special qualities required in an effective crisis responder.

Debriefer Characteristics

Available	Mentally tough
Independent	Hides one's own ego
Team player	Can do outreach
Takes orders	Action junkie
Uses support	Physically strong
Does not know everything	Able to camp out
Egalitarian	

The goals, and therefore the training, of the immediate responders to disaster are specific and focused on the needs of the survivors. Immediate disaster response is not therapy in its traditional sense and definition. The goal of immediate response is to return power and control to the survivors, which precludes probing and judgmental attitudes. For long-term care, a thorough and focused understanding of PTSD is necessary.

Although the focus on trauma survivors, victims, and their needs has a relatively short history, the pioneers wisely recognized the need for special training almost immediately. By 1989, the ISTSS had developed a comprehensive curriculum resource for PTSD education. The vigorous and rapid expansion of this field dictated that new opportunities for special training continue to be developed.

Established training programs include those for military personnel who participate in Massive Casualty Exercise Training and learn to respond to simulated disasters. For civilians, the Red Cross, with offices in most major cities, offers basic disaster training and multiple advanced training courses which include attention to natural disasters. The National Organization for Victim Assistance (NOVA) offers the National Crisis Response Team Training Institute, an intensive forty-hour residential training which provides a certificate of recognition to those who successfully complete the course. The participant's manual offered is continually updated. Retraining to update participant skills and knowledge is recommended at least every two years. Tom Williams offers a two-day training course by arrangement and as an invited conference presenter. Jeffrey Mitchell, with the International Critical Debriefing Society, has provided training focused on peer debriefing in the United States and internationally for many years.

The International Association of Trauma Counselors (IATC) offers a Certified Trauma Counselor/Specialist Certificate to those who successfully fulfill its requirements for both specific trauma didactic education and for supervised experience. In addition, the IATC issues certificates of Associate in Trauma Response (ATR) for those specifically trained for natural disaster response. Since 1992, in affiliation with IATC, the Jersey City State College Institute for Trauma Studies has offered approved courses applicable towards certification by IATC. This Institute was the result of extensive efforts by Shelley Neiderbach, chairperson of the IATC Education and Training Task Force. Due to budgetary constraints, this institute was closed in 1995.

At the University of Wisconsin, Chris Dunning, PhD, has developed a teaching program on trauma that is offered to other degree-granting institutions. These training opportunities are some examples of a rapidly expanding education area, but are not meant to be an exhaustive nor comprehensive list. Simply stated, in extraordinary circumstance, as after a natural disaster, training beyond the ordinary is required. Fortunately, for the survivors of catastrophe special training opportunities are available.

I have learned this: It is not what one does that is wrong,
but what one becomes as a consequence of it.

Oscar Wilde

ACUTE TRAUMA DEBRIEFING

Joel Osler Brende, MD

Acute trauma debriefing or critical incident debriefing refers to those interventions which are designed to quickly help trauma survivors with their emotional distress to preclude the onset of protected Post-traumatic symptoms. Debriefing is particularly useful with large groups of survivors following natural disasters, industrial mishaps, community disasters, accidents involving aircraft or multiple vehicles and violent or unexpected deaths involving noted individuals and community or organizational leaders. Debriefing may take place as a primary intervention at the scene, as secondary, away from the scene or tertiary, shortly afterwards, preferably within 24-48 hours. In some cases, survivors may require follow-up counseling or therapy.

Debriefing interventions provide a systematized approach similar to that which most sensitive parents instinctively use at times of their children's' distressful moments. When five year-old Johnny comes home from the playground with skin abrasions and torn clothing, crying profusely, his mother immediately intervenes with a hug. After his sobs have abated, Johnny's mother asks what happened. As he stumbles through a description of the traumatic event, she listens empathically, finds out what is seriously wrong, what is not, and takes appropriate action for medical care if necessary. Although Johnny may feel guilty about having been in a fight with another playmate, his mother listens and assures him of her love. Finally, she assures his that is he wakes up and has a bad dream that night, she will be there to reassure him. With all of this support, Johnny will feel better both physically and emotionally, although he may talk about the incident again, at bedtime, and in the future.

Johnny's mother provided the essentials of debriefing: 1) Clarification: to help the survivor clarify and identify the events that occurred; 2) Expression: to provide an opportunity for emotional catharsis within the context of a loving and supportive environment; 3) Education: provision of information about normal responses and potential symptoms that may later develop; 4) Restoration: provision of hope and plans for the future.

Debriefing is important, not only to prevent long-standing Post-traumatic symptoms, but to enable something more positive to occur. For example, Johnny's

161

traumatic experience, without the loving intervention of his mother, might have resulted in shame, distrust, persistent fear, and anger. Instead, because of an empathic listener and the provision of education and hope, the experience had a strengthening effect on the development of his character while enhancing a reservoir of ego coping skills.

Who should use debriefing principles and techniques? Although they are often instinctively used by parents and friends, these skills can easily be taught to any interested individual. Debriefing principles should be learned by professionals such as medical personnel, mental health counselors, pastoral counselors and selected paraprofessionals. But, beyond that, because of the preponderance of traumatic events in this country and worldwide, debriefing principles and techniques should be taught to relief workers and interested volunteers from helping organizations and churches.

What if debriefing is not available or does not work? There are times when debriefing may not be provided, may not be adequate, or the trauma could be excessively horrendous. Unfortunately, there are many victims who do not have access to debriefing or who maintain secrecy about their traumatic experiences. Sexual assault victims, victims of violent crime, and witnesses to violent acts often are not adequately debriefed. Because of the lack of opportunity, or lack of available and caring debriefers, these survivors remain burdened with shame, anger, fear or distrust and are predisposed to become re-victimized at some later time in their lives. Unfortunately, the escalation of violent crime and other kinds of traumatic events, within this country and worldwide, is creating an environment for mushrooming victimization and increasing the numbers of victims with residual Post-traumatic symptoms.

Debriefing is essential. When it is not available or when survivors required a longer period of time for recovery, there are other avenues of help available. For those who need more than what debriefing can accomplish, follow-up support groups, psychotherapy, and psycho-educational groups are recommended (Brende, 1994). Fortunately, the self-help group movement in this country has also spread into the arena of supporting victims and survivors. For those who are interested, the author has developed a unique twelve theme and step program which is available for professional and self-help group use (Brende, 1990, 1991, 1992, 1993). A summary of those twelve themes is described below:

TWELVE THEMES AND RECOVERY STEPS FOR VICTIMS

1. Power vs. Victimization

Do you find yourself repeatedly victimized and seem to have no power to break the cycle? If so, accept that you are powerless, ask for help from someone willing to help you, and consider the possibility that there is also a Higher Power from whom you can seek help.

2. Seeking Meaning

Are you confused and believe your life has no meaning? If so, seek a source of meaning for your life and look for help to do so, from your Higher Power, God, as you individually understand God to be.

3. Trust vs. Shame and Doubt

Do you feel bad, ashamed and distrusting? If so, find someone you can trust, someone to whom you can begin to talk, share, be yourself, and seek to trust your Higher Power.

4. Self-Inventory

Do you feel detached, indifferent, or deny you have any kind of a problem? If so, be open to the truth from someone you trust and from your Higher Power. Ask yourself these questions: Do I do things that hurt myself or others? Do I need to change something in my life? What steps must I take in order to change?

5. Anger

Do you become angry in ways that are destructive? If so, learn how to control your destructive anger, and assert yourself in positive ways with help from someone you trust and your Higher Power.

6. Fear

Have you become unduly frightened, phobic or paranoid, or do you take unnecessary, dangerous risks? If so, understand the nature of healthy fear, but find ways to resolve your excessive fear and dangerous risk-taking with help from someone you trust and your Higher Power.

7. Guilt

Do you feel overwhelmed with guilt, or have you lost your conscience, sensitivity, and sense of responsibility for your actions? If so, seek the forgiveness of those you have hurt, if possible, and then forgive yourself with help from someone you trust and your Higher Power.

8. Grief

Are you grieving excessively, depressed or alienated from others? If so, grieve for whomever or whatever you have lost and seek to regain your capacity to cry and experience joy, with the help of someone you trust and your Higher Power.

9. Life vs. Death

Are you self-destructive, suicidal, or addicted? If so, seek justice for your grievances, but then relinquish your bitterness, learn how to laugh at your situation and make a commitment to learn how to forgive, with help from someone you trust and your Higher Power.

10. Justice vs. Revenge

Are you bitter, hostile, or do you often hurt other people? If so seek justice for your grievances, but then relinquish your bitterness, learn how to laugh at your situation and make a commitment to learn how to forgive - with help from someone you trust and your Higher Power.

11. Finding a Purpose

Have you become unduly fanatical or have episodes when you become unpredictable? If so, seek a proper balance in your life, a purpose for your life, and a personal relationship with your Higher Power, while learning how to laugh at yourself.

12. Love and Relationships

Are you enslaved in a destructive situation, in prison or incarcerated? If so, seek liberation from your slavery through acceptance of the love and leadership of your Higher Power.

If you are a victim, follow these aforementioned recovery steps and you have an excellent opportunity to develop a new pattern of living which will break your particular victimization cycle. Take them one step and one day at a time.

Chaos demands to be recognized and experienced
before letting itself be converted into a new order.

Hermann Hesse

COUNTERTRANSFERENCE AND TRAINING

Yael Danieli, PhD

The last two decades have witnessed a growing recognition of the effects, sometimes lasting, on caregivers during and in the aftermath of disasters. Accordingly, various measures have been developed to psychologically inoculate them. The exercise process described below is one such attempt, originally generated to train therapists working with Holocaust survivors and their children and later used to work through other *event countertransferences.*

BACKGROUND

The phrase *conspiracy of silence* has been used to describe the typical interaction of Holocaust survivors and their children with psychotherapists when Holocaust experiences were mentioned or recounted (Krystal & Niederland, 1968), as it has been used to portray their interaction with society in general. Whereas, society has a moral obligation to share its members' pain, psychotherapists and researchers have, in addition, a professional contractual obligation. When they fail to listen, explore, understand, and help, they too inflict the "trauma after the trauma" (Rappaport, 1968), or "The 'Second Injury' to Victims" (Symonds, 1980) by maintaining and perpetuating the *conspiracy of silence.*

Elsewhere, this author has reviewed in detail the literature on the conspiracy of silence (Danieli, 1982a), described its harmful long-term impact on the survivors (Danieli, 1994d), their families (1981a, 1985) and their psychotherapists (Danieli, 1988) and reported research on therapists' difficulties in treating survivors of the Nazi Holocaust and their children (Danieli, 1982a, 1988). The later research identified and examined 49 countertransference reactions and attitudes reported in the literature and by 61 psychotherapists working with survivors and children of survivors of the Nazi Holocaust.

In order of frequency, some of the major categories of countertransference phenomena systematically examined in the study were *various modes of defense* against listening to Holocaust experiences and against therapists' inability to

165

contain their intense emotional reactions (e.g., numbing, denial, avoidance, distancing, clinging to professional role, reduction to method and/or theory); *affective reactions* such as bystander's guilt, rage, with its variety of objects, dread and horror, shame and related emotions (e.g., disgust and loathing), grief and mourning; "me too," sense of bond, privileged voyeurism, and specific *relational context issues* such as parent-child relationship, victim/liberator, viewing the survivor as hero, and attention and attitudes toward Jewish identity. These themes are reported, described, illustrated, and discussed in detail in a series of articles elsewhere (Danieli, 1980, 1982a, 1984, 1988, 1994a, 1994b).

The fact that 18 of the 61 psychotherapists in the original study were themselves survivors and children of survivors of the Nazi Holocaust permitted a comparison between their reactions and those of the participants who were not. This data is reported fully in Danieli (1982a),and partially in Danieli (1988), and will not be described here because of space limitations. However, one could look for parallels of differing responses in terms of reactions of caregivers who are members of the communities effected by disaster and those who are not, including the often-reported "onslaught of outside helpers and reporters" and "imported projects."

COUNTERTRANSFERENCE IN TRAINING PROFESSIONALS WORKING WITH TRAUMA

Traditional training generally has not prepared professionals to deal with *massive real trauma* and its long-term effects. In-house, on-the-job-site training supervision has been offered by various agencies. The ISTSS has begun to ameliorate this lack of training, among other activities, through its Initial Report from the 1989 Presidential Task Force on Curriculum, Education and Training (Danieli and Krystal, 1989). This report contains model curricula formulated by leading international specialists in the field and is composed of subcommittees representing different technical specialties or interests including psychiatry, psychology, social work, nursing, creative arts therapy, clergy and media, organizations, institutions and public health, paraprofessionals and other professionals, and undergraduate education. The need to recognize, cope with, and work through countertransference difficulties was seen as imperative for optimal training in this field.

As early as 1980 (Danieli, 1980), with the published preliminary thematic overview of the above mentioned study, it was stated that, "While this cluster [of countertransference reactions] was reported by professionals working with Jewish Holocaust survivors and their offspring, this author believes that other victim/survivor populations may be responded to similarly and may suffer similar [consequences]. Defining the[se] reaction-clusters ... will lead therapists and investigators to be better able to recognize them so that they can monitor, contain and use them preventively and therapeutically." In 1981 it was noted that these reactions "seem very similar to alexithymia, anhedonia, and their concomitants and components which, according to Krystal, characterize survivors" (Danieli, 1981b). In 1989, in the context of training (Danieli, 1981b), these phenomena were referred to as the "vicarious victimization of the caregiver."

These insights and hypotheses about the ubiquity of countertransference reactions in other victim populations have now moved to the forefront of our concern in the preparation and training of professionals who work with victims and trauma survivors. Indeed, the ensuing literature reflected a growing realization among professionals working with other victims/survivors of the need to describe, understand and organize different elements and aspects of the *conspiracy of silence* (Danieli, 1994a, 1994b; Dyregrov & Mitchell, 1992; Herman, 1992; Wilson & Lindy, 1994). Countertransference reactions are integral ubiquitous and expected.

Our work calls on us to confront, with our patients and within ourselves, extraordinary human experiences. This confrontation is profoundly humbling in that at all times these experiences try our view of the world we live in and challenge the limits of our humanity.

In reality, countertransference reactions are the building blocks of the societal as well as professional *conspiracy of silence*. They inhibit professionals from studying, correctly diagnosing and treating the effects of trauma. They also perpetuate the heretofore pervasive absence of traditional training necessary for professionals to cope with *massive (adult) real trauma* and its long-term effects.

Although information cannot undo unconscious reactions, knowledge about trauma in their historic context does provide the therapist with a factual and, for example, gender, ethnic, racial, religious, cultural, or political perspectives that help him or her know what to look for, what may be missing in the survivor's account of his or her experience(s), and what types of questions to ask. But, countertransference reactions interfere in the process of acquiring the knowledge about the trauma as well (Danieli, 1994a).

In addition to information about the trauma terrain, familiarity with the growing body of literature on the long-term psychological sequelae of the trauma on the survivors and their offspring also helps prepare mental health professionals. Nonetheless, they should guard against the simple grouping of individuals as "survivors," and expect all of them to exhibit the same "survivor syndrome" (Krystal & Niederland, 1968), or PTSD.

Many of the countertransference phenomena examined were found to be reactions to patient's Holocaust *stories* rather than to their behavior. The unusual uniformity of psychotherapists' reactions suggests that they are in response to the

Holocaust, the one fact that all the otherwise different patients have in common. Because the Holocaust seems to be the source of these reactions, it is suggested that it is appropriate to name them *countertransference reactions to the Holocaust,* rather than to the patients themselves. I also believe that therapists' difficulties in treating other victim/survivor populations may similarly have their roots in the nature of their victimization *(event countertransference).*

PROCESSING EVENT COUNTERTRANSFERENCE

Regarding event countertransferences as dimensions of the inner, or *intrapsychic, conspiracy of silence* about the trauma allows us the possibility to explore and confront these reactions to the trauma events prior to and independent of the therapeutic encounter with the victim/survivor patient, in a variety of training and supervisory settings and by ourselves. Presented below is an exercise process developed over the last two decades which has been proven helpful in numerous workshops, training institutes, debriefing of "front liners," seminars, and in consultative, supervisory relationships around the world, to work through *event countertransference.* While it originally evolved, and is still done optimally, as a part of a group experience, it can also be done alone and assist the clinician working privately. As one veteran traumatologist who uses it regularly stated, "It is like taking an inner shower when I am stuck with...[a] patient..."

INSTRUCTIONS FOR PARTICIPANTS

In a group setting, participants are asked to arrange the chairs in a circle. (Participants can be trauma caregivers, trauma survivors, and/or both). After everyone is seated, without any introductions, they're told, "Take a large piece of paper, a pen or a pencil. Create space for yourself. The first phase of the process will be private totally between you and yourself." If in group setting: "Please, don't talk with each other during this first phase."

"Choose the victimization/trauma experience most meaningful to you." This author always begins with the Holocaust, and after completing the total process described below about the Holocaust, only then are the participants asked to take another large piece of paper and to choose the victimization/trauma experience most meaningful to them. Facilitators may modify the event countertransference they choose as a starting point for this exercise to optimize the process in their own situation. "Please, let yourself focus in on it."

1. **Imaging:** Draw everything and anything, any image that comes to mind when you think about the experience you chose. Take your time. We have a lot of time. Take all the time you need.

2. **Word Association:** When you have completed this task, turn the page, and please, write down every word that comes to mind when you focus on this experience.

3. **Added Reflection and Affective Associations:** When you finish this, draw a line underneath the words. Please, look through/reflect on the words you have written. Is there any effect or feeling word that you may have not included? Please, add them now. Roam freely around you mind, and add any other word that comes to mind now.

4. **First Memory:** When was the very *first time* you ever heard of ___, the very first time. How did you hear? What was it like for you? Who did you hear it from? Or what did you hear it from? Go back and explore that situation in your mind with as much detail as you can: What was it like? How old were you? Where are you in the memory? Are you in the kitchen, in the bedroom, living room, in class, in the movies, in the park? Are you watching TV? Are you alone or with other people? Who? With your parents, family, friends? What are you feeling? Do you remember any particular physical sensations? What are you thinking?

5. **Choices and Beliefs:** Are you making any *choices* about life, about people, about yourself at the time of the memory. Decisions like:
   "Because this happened, therefore ...," or
   "This means that life is ...,
   that people are ...,
   that the world is ..."
   What are you telling yourself, are you coming to any conclusions? This is very important. Stay with that.

6. **Continuity and Discontinuity of Self:** Think of yourself today, look at that situation, are you still holding those choices? Do you still believe what you concluded then? Would you say "this is still me" or, "this is not me anymore"? What is the difference, what changed and why?

7. **Sharing with others:** Have you *talked with other* people about it? Who did you talk to? Both in the past and present. What was their reaction? What was you reaction to their reaction?

8. **Secrets: Not Sharing with Others:** If there is anything about this that you haven't told anyone, that you decided that it is not to be talked about, that it's "unspeakable"? Is there any area in it that you feel that is totally your *secret*, that you dealt with all alone and kept to yourself? If there is, please put it into words such as, "I haven't shared it because...," or, "I am very hesitant to share it because..." Would you please mention the particular people with whom you won't share it, and why.

9. **Personal Knowledge of Survivors:** Moving to another aspect, of the *interpersonal realm,* do you personally know survivors of___or their family members, as friends, neighbors or colleagues?

10. **Self-Secrets:** There are secrets we keep from others to protect either ourselves or them, and there are *self-secrets.* Take your time. This is very important. Imagine the situation of the very first time you ever heard anything about it. Roam inside your mind. Is there anything about it that you have never talked to yourself about, a secret you have kept from yourself? An area that you have sort of pushed away or kept at arms length from yourself? Or about which you say to yourself, "I can't handle that?" Why is it the one thing that was too much for you? What haven't you put into words yet, that is still lurking in that corner of your mind you have not looked into yet?

11. **Personal Relationship to the Trauma:** What is your *personal relationship* to the trauma? Please, do write the answers, because even the way you write makes a difference. Did your place of birth figure in your relationship to the trauma? Does your age figure in your relationship to the trauma?

12. **Identity Dimensions:** What is your *religious, ethnic, cultural, political, class, racial and gender* identity? Do these parts of your identity figure in the choices you made, influence your relationship to the experience? How? You can answer these one by one.

13. **Professional Relationship to the Trauma:** Let us move to your *professional* self, what is your professional discipline? How long have you been working in it? Your discipline? What is your professional relationship to the trauma? Within your professional practice, have you seen survivors of___? Or their children of___? How many?

14. **Therapeutic Orientation:** What therapeutic modality did you employ? Emergency/crisis intervention, short, long-term, individual, family, and/or group therapy? Was it in an inpatient or outpatient basis? What modality have you found most useful, and why?

15. **Victim and Trauma Survivor Populations:** Was it the only victim/survivor population you have worked with professionally?

16. **Training in Trauma Work:** Have you ever been trained to work with victim/survivors of trauma? In school, on the job? If you were, what have you found to be the crucial elements of your training without which you won't feel prepared to do the job?

The sequence in the first phase of processing the event countertransference is from the immediate visual imagery, through free associations to the more verbal-cognitive material. It then moves to articulate how the trauma fits within the therapist's experience, personal and interpersonal development and the gender, racial, ethnic, religious, cultural and political realms of her or his life. It begins with one's *private* world of trauma and proceeds through the context of one's interpersonal life to one's professional work.

While the material can be analyzed privately, the second phase of the process, the sharing and exploring phase, works best in a group setting, as is often the case with survivors and children of survivors of the Nazi Holocaust (Danieli, 1988; 1989) and with other victims/survivors. As with trauma survivors, therapists are able to explore with each other, comprehend the consequences in their lives of the trauma they have experienced directly or indirectly and the conspiracy of silence that frequently follows them, and share their feelings and concerns. The group modality thus serves to counteract their own sense of isolation and alienation about working with trauma.

Elsewhere, in discussing the value of the group modalities for the victim/survivor patients, this author suggested that groups have been particularly helpful in compensating for countertransference reactions. Whereas a therapist alone may feel unable to contain or provide a "holding environment" (Winnicott, 1965) for his or her patient's feelings, the group as a unit is able to do this. While any particularly intense interaction invoked by trauma memories may prove too overwhelming to some people present, others invariably come forth with a variety of helpful "holding" reactions. Thus, the group functions as an ideal absorptive entity for abreaction and catharsis of emotions, especially negative ones, that are otherwise experienced as uncontainable. Finally, the group modality offers a multiplicity of options for expressing, naming, verbalizing and modulating feelings. It provides a safe place for exploring fantasies, for imagining, "inviting," and taking on the roles and examining their significance in the identity of the participants. Finally, the group encourages and demonstrates mutual support and caring, which ultimately enhances self-care. These considerations apply to therapists working in groups as well.

This training process assumes that the most meaningful way to tap into event countertransferences is to let them emerge, in a systematic way, from the particularity of the therapist's experience. She or he can thus be better able to recognize and become familiar with her or his own reactions in order to monitor, and learn to understand and contain them, as well as use them preventively and therapeutically. During the sharing phase, when participants describe the images they drew and the process of selecting them, they already put them into words.

Space does not permit describing the richness of what can be learned in on-going, prolonged group supervision processes. The interacting tapestries of, among others, event countertransference and person countertransference, the mutual impact of differing adaptational styles to the trauma (Danieli, 1985) of therapists and patients, examination of mutual (counter)transferences among members are played out in the group dynamics. One important instance of the latter is the attempted expulsion of the supervisor, the person leading the exercise process, who thus becomes the symbolic agent of the trauma, from the group for "victimizing" them and exposing their vulnerabilities by encouraging them to confront, (re)experience, the trauma.

The exercise incurs ambivalence as well. Claiming an inability to draw, and a preference to "only do the words part" is an obvious example of resistance. The exercise process does not aim to replace ongoing supervisory countertransference work. It does, however, aim to provide a sorely needed focus on and an experiential multidimensional framework for the trauma aspects of the patients' and therapists' lives.

The process also helps build awareness of the caregiver's vulnerability to being vicariously victimized (McCann & Pearlman, 1990) by repeated exposure to trauma and trauma stories and to the toll countertransference reactions take on intrapsychic, interpersonal and family lives.

The exercise process poignantly makes clear the paramount necessity of careful nurturing, regulating and ensuring the development of a self-protective, self-healing and self-soothing way of being as a professional and a full human being. The importance of self-care and self-soothing is acknowledged in the exercise in building into the process instructional elements such as "take your time...take all the time you need," and a caring, respectful attention to every element explored. Although not included in the above version of the exercise, special effort is made to include soothing, supportive instructional language.

The composition of the workshop or seminar group may be unpredictable. One can be assured, however, that many of the psychotherapists present have been themselves, directly or indirectly, victims or trauma survivors, whose victimization either inspired and energized their choice of work/career or specialty, or interacts with their patient's trauma as part of their countertransference matrix. Invariably, also, group members learn about cultures other than their own. They come to finish unfinished business with their patients and with themselves, to explore their wounds, clean the pus, and to heal. They come to seek answers, to find forgiveness and compassion and ultimately, understanding and camaraderie. They mobilize creative energy and allow themselves to transform as people to be more authentic in their work and more actualized in their personal lives.

SOME PRINCIPLES OF SELF HEALING

The following principles are designed to help professionals recognize, contain and heal *event countertransferences*.

A. To recognize own reactions:
   1. Develop awareness of somatic signals of distress - one's chart of warning signs of potential countertransference reaction, e.g., sleeplessness, headaches, perspiration.

2. Try to find words to name accurately and to articulate one's inner experiences and feelings. As Bettelheim (1984) commented, "what cannot be talked about can also not be put to rest; and if it is not, the wounds continue to fester from generation to generation" (pg. 166).

B. To contain own reactions:
1. Identify a personal level of comfort in order to build openness, tolerance and readiness to hear anything.
2. Knowing that every emotion has a beginning, a middle and an end, learn to attenuate the fear of being overwhelmed by its intensity to try to feel its full life-cycle without resorting to defensive countertransference reactions.

C. To heal and grow:
1. Accept that nothing will ever be the same.
2. When wounded, one should take time, accurately diagnose, soothe and heal before being "emotionally fit" again to continue to work.
3. Seek consultation or further therapy for previously unexplored areas triggered by patients' stories.
4. Any one of the affective reactions (i.e., grief, mourning, rage) may interact with *old, unresolved* experiences of the therapists. They will thus be able to use their professional work purposefully for their own growth. One survivor of a childhood trauma, mother and psychotherapist, through further integration of her insights and understanding, was able to turn her vulnerability into a source of sensitivity and strength. She was able to help her patients, and also enrich and deepen her relationships with her husband and children.
5. Establish a network of people to create a holding environment (Winnicot, 1965) within which one can share one's trauma-related work (Danieli, 1994c).
6. Therapists should provide themselves with avocational avenues for creative and relaxing self-expression in order to regenerate energies.
   Being kind to oneself and feeling free to have fun and joy is not a frivolity in this field but a necessity without which professional obligations, professional contracts cannot be fulfilled.

It is extraordinary how
extraordinary the ordinary person is.

George F. Will

FOSTERING RESILIENCY IN DISASTER RESPONDERS

Chris Dunning, PhD

Contrary to depictions of trauma responders portrayed on television and in other media, disaster mitigation professionals do not generally respond to traumatic events with role conflict, panic or shock. Rescuers rarely disintegrate or become incapable of performing and coping during and subsequent to the disaster. Acute-stress and/or Post-traumatic reactions do not suddenly appear within minutes or hours in the overwhelming majority of disaster personnel (Dunning & Silva, 1981).

People responding to the professional demands of a disastrous situation do what they have to do to survive, to protect themselves and others and to rescue those who may be in need of immediate aid. They invest their efforts in disaster intervention and mitigation. Responders involved in traumatic situations do not generally become panic-stricken, dissociative or ineffective. They have a great capacity to think and act, to respond to and resolve traumatic events even in the face of great risk and horror. This is not to say, however, that emotional and behavioral problems do not frequently surface later among responders. These problems, varying in nature, intensity and duration, may affect the quality of life and professional performance of disaster responders. It is important to note that not all the effects of trauma are negative, however. Some of the positive effects of trauma are enhancement or reinforcement of the responder's ability to cope with adversity, self-discipline, appreciation for the value of life, and a sense of accomplishment, competence, assertiveness and resilience.

Mistaken ideas about mental health problems that may occur after a trauma persist despite empirical data that suggest otherwise. Only a small minority of emergency workers experience severe stress, much less an acute or Post-traumatic stress reaction following deployment in an emergency situation. On average, studies of emergency workers have found that approximately 2% to 17% of such workers develop Post-traumatic sequelae. Admonitions such as "You must be debriefed or you will experience PTSD or something just as dire" are commonly heard by disaster workers. The reality, however, is that such statements are

174

exaggerations. In fact, the few studies of the impact of debriefing on the subsequent development of Post-traumatic symptoms would suggest the opposite, that in fact debriefing exacerbates traumatic stress given the increased number of diagnosed PTSD among the debriefed (Meichenbaum, 1994). Most emergency workers don't suffer traumatic stress but rather mild and moderate stress, which in fact is a completely different physiological phenomenon. In fact what studies of debriefing should be addressing is a reduction in stress as opposed to traumatic stress, which is a neurobiological phenomena involving different physiological, endrocrinological, and neurological reactions than stress. In addition, since approximately 77% of all persons suffering acute stress and Post-traumatic stress reactions spontaneously go into remission within six months subsequent to the trauma without any intervention (Breslau et al., 1992), it is difficult to point to debriefing as having a salutary effect on traumatic stress.

One can argue that we have been too quick to grab the first technique that presents itself as having an impact in problematic behavior (Davidson, 1979; Dunning and Silva, 1980; Wagner, 1981; Mantell, 1984). Talk therapy has been the mainstay of psychological treatment. To have done something, such as debriefing, where nothing was done before in response to a need brings with it the satisfaction and cognitive dissonance so frequently experienced by pioneers. The reality, however, is that for something as complex and pervasive as trauma, one therapeutic approach is hardly adequate or acceptable to assist traumatized persons to recover. In fact, despite market surveys presented as empirical research, which ask the client how much they benefited from or felt the debriefing helped, debriefing has not shown itself to address or ameliorate the deleterious consequences of responding to disaster for some workers. Expressions of irritation at having been required to participate in debriefing or perceptions that it is a waste of time are common. That is not to say that here has not been workers who truly believe that debriefing has been helpful.

It is important that any formal response subsequent to a traumatic event build upon the strengths and capabilities of the responders. Disaster responders are normal persons, who are generally capable of functioning in an effective manner, both physically and emotionally. These professionals have been subjected to severe stress and it is not unusual that they may show signs of emotional strain. This transitory disturbance is to be expected and does not necessarily imply mental illness or Post-traumatic reaction.

The most difficult of responses to trauma that result in post-event intervention involve the themes of meaning (Hedrman, 1992), imagery, and control. Yet debriefing does not specifically address these areas, focusing instead on normalization of affect, physical symptomatology, and the development of social contracts. It would appear that it is time, now that we have "OWNED" the idea of traumatic stress in emergency work that we begin to expand our understanding and develop new intervention strategies that would support emergency workers.

DEVELOPING A DISASTER TRAUMA RECOVERY THEORY

Figley, in his book, *Healing Traumatized Families* (1989), speaks to the need of the family to develop a healing theory in order to recover from trauma. Such an approach is also useful in considering how to maintain an emergency worker during and subsequent to development at a traumatic event. We have generated a new expectation in emergency work, that disaster deployment leads inevitably to PTSD unless debriefed or otherwise treated. The "theory" being espoused suggests not one of improvement, but of decline. It would appear that the experience of disaster deployment is currently being perceived as being the basis for pathology, focusing on emotional wounds and psychiatric casualties.

In order to maintain the integrity of the disaster worker, it would seem advantageous to develop a response that would not automatically use a *sickness* or *pathogenic* model (Antonovky, 1979, 1986, 1990a, 1990b, 1990c, 1991, 1993) aimed at dealing with the worker's perceived present or future "emotional problems." Just as it is inappropriate to treat workers as needing rescuing, saving or protection before demonstrated need, one should not assume that an inevitable consequence of disaster deployment will be PTSD, or sickness. As mentioned previously, disaster workers do not disintegrate in response to trauma. They have an immediate need to feel as if they are still in control in a situation that is out of control. For the most part, workers respond amazingly well to traumatic situations considering the amount of stress they may have endured. Feelings of helplessness, caused by the event itself, will only be aggravated if mental health professionals reinforce the perception that the worker needs to turn control over to a "debriefer" in order to survive the disaster experience. This is contrary to Figley's conception of a healing theory, which supports resilience and expectation of future accomplishment over the travails caused by the event.

Being based on a pathogenic model, debriefing has its roots in the theoretical orientations of learned helplessness. Behaviorally-oriented psychologists assume that maladaptive behaviors are produced and maintained by environmental contingencies, hence traumatic events lead to the behaviors of the traumatized. Cognitively-oriented psychologists believe that mental disorders originate from irrational beliefs and 'cognitive distortions.' What each shares in common is the pathogenic model (Rosenbaum, 1990). Antonovsky (1987) argues for the abandonment of the pathogenic model in favor of the salutogenic model which focuses on the cultural, social, and personal resources that contribute to successful coping and mental health. This orientation is similar to Meichenbaum's

176

(1985) Stress Inoculation Training (SIT), which was designed to nurture and develop coping skills or "learned resourcefulness." Learned resourcefulness refers to what one can do when stressful circumstances call for self-direction. Antonovsky's sense of coherence furthers this concept to include a set of personal beliefs that guide the way with which one copes with stress. A sense of coherence expresses the belief that life, or the situation at hand, is comprehensible, manageable, and meaningful.

It is more appropriate and effective to follow a wellness or salutogenic model that focuses on supporting the worker in retaining control. Disaster workers need to be provided with support and information. Many workers are unable to accept, and will even actively refuse help if they surmise that in your eyes they are injured or mentally disordered. Disaster counselors who assume the worst case scenario alienate disaster workers. Just because an individual has experienced a traumatic event does not necessarily mean that he or she requires mental health intervention. The establishment of a system of triage is often overlooked in trauma mental health response for disaster workers as is the possibilities that are afforded by acting as a psychological consultant to administration. The trigger for offering services tends to be the experience of a traumatic event rather than a rational assessment of the individual's need for services. The debriefing acts as the response of the organization to the traumatic event, what Mantell (1984) and Dunning (1988) call a "band-aid" approach to dealing with work-related mental injuries.

It is the fear of affect overload that makes most disaster workers wary of offers of psychological counseling. The worker who is particularly traumatized may have established a fragile equilibrium that may be threatened by talk of the event or its mental injury potential. Because traumatized persons may go through a denial phase in response to a traumatic event, offers of counseling may be rebuffed and mandatory attempts to render assistance prove useless. Workers report being overwhelmed in debriefing sessions, adding the imagery and story reported by others into their own traumatic "set," thus increasing the troubling issues of control, imagery, and meaning. Instead of helping the worker to resolve the traumatic incident by putting words to images, the universe of both words and images are expanded, confabulated, and adapted. The worker can be overwhelmed by the enormity of the event, burdened by the damage reported by others, and feel helpless that the event can ever be resolved. We are asking the disaster worker, in participating in a group debrief, to shoulder the injuries and experiences of others at a time in which workers who are truly traumatized have already reached their 'limit,' their ability to tolerate traumatic material.

Most traditional clinical intervention strategies used in mental health treatment are not appropriate when working with acutely traumatized persons. Behaviors that the therapist may see as pathological or maladaptive in fact may be appropriate and adaptive for the worker, given his or her traumatic experience.

Denial serves people well in the short run if they must face grotesque scenes of horror in order to resolve crisis situations and rescue workers. A numb or dampened affect may assist the worker to re-establish a sense of safety and support, the behaviors necessary for survival and action. Everstine and Everstine (1993) conclude that traditional approaches of treatment and crisis intervention are not appropriate to acute trauma in that these approaches presuppose a higher level of intellectual functioning than people who have been recently traumatized can muster. The reflective technique of crisis intervention strategies employs a level of abstraction and cognitive reasoning that is beyond the acutely traumatized person. The Everstines suggest that the reflective approach only adds to the fears and frustrations of a person whose thinking is impaired. In fact, to encourage a traumatized person to think analytically may result in the person becoming more anxious, confused or to 'shut down.'

Additionally, methods designed to induce catharsis are generally not recommended for use immediately following a trauma experience. Everstine and Everstine (1993) posit that it is not conducive to recovery to encourage a traumatized person to 'let go of' or 'vent' feelings at a time when the person is struggling to regain composure and to make sense of chaos, horror or loss. The Everstines point out that clinicians need to be aware that emotions may be the only thing the traumatized person feels he or she can control. Any cathartic response elicited - - crying, screaming, story telling - - may not provide psychological relief to the person. It is questionable whether persons who experience dissociative reactions during disaster work benefit from debriefing. The surreal experiences of derealization and depersonalization are so upsetting to the internal locus of control of the rescue worker that to divulge their occurrence would not only be seen as "professional suicide" but would not be realistic in the group process generated by a debrief. In this case, the worker is left to believe that they are really "going crazy" as dissociate experiences other than the "thousand-yard stare" are rarely discussed. What surfaces in debriefing in both the educational and psychological components are *acceptable* sequelae such as nightmares and sleep disturbances, not the realities of the acutely stressed. For that reason, debriefing might serve well for stress reactions but not for acute or Post-traumatic stress by invoking a pathological approach.

The wellness or salutogenic approach to serving the mental health needs of disaster workers incorporates research and theory on hardiness and resiliency. Hardiness represents the ability of an individual to become inured to fatigue or hardship, and to be capable of withstanding austere or horrific conditions (Funk, 1992). It is a worker's resolute courage and fortitude in the face of the overwhelming demands occasioned by the disastrous event (Williams et al., 1992). Hardiness is thought to represent the characteristic manner in which a person approaches and interprets an experience (Bartone et al., 1989). It is described variously along the five dimensions noted below, with the attributes of control, challenge and commitment significantly influencing how people process and cope with stressful events (Kobasa et al., 1982).

Resiliency involves the capability of recovery after stress or to adjust to dramatic changes. The personality style of hardiness (dispositional resiliency) has been shown to have a moderating effect on traumatic stress symptoms (Bartone et al., 1989). Anatonsvsky (1993) first posited that a salutogenic orientation versus a pathogenic orientation has far wider implications than simply proving a directive to focus on the health rather than the pathology of traumatized persons. According to Antonovsky (1987, 1990, 1990b), a "sense of coherence," or way of making sense of the world, is a major factor in determining how well a person manages stress and stays healthy. This is in some ways similar to the treatise of Janoff-Bulman in *Shattered Assumptions* (1992) and the meaning discussed by Herman in *Trauma and Recovery* (1992). Antonovsky suggested that the neurophysiological, endocrinological, and immunological pathways through which the sense of coherence operates influences health outcomes that are associated with traumatic events (1990c).

THE TASKS OF WELLNESS

Using a wellness approach to trauma counseling, the trauma counselor in the acute stage of trauma should assess the previous coping skills of the worker as well as assess their resiliency and hardiness. Following Maddi and Kobasa's (1984) hardiness approach to stress is particularly functional in the initial, post-trauma counseling session subsequent to the education noted above.

The tasks to be performed at the acute stage of disaster (trans-or immediately post-event) include:

1. *Control:* learning to gain mastery over symptomatology and support empowerment to gain control over situation, activities, etc. This may represent attempts at cognitive control which may involve beginning to think differently about the disaster and ensuing response and its implications. Persons requiring this type of control need a sounding board for discussion of the event, and analyses of their role and actions in the event. Some might seek to change the circumstances through direct action such as resigning, asking for transfer, or volunteering for overtime assignment on the disaster site, etc. This type of person seeks activities and actions that enhance their sense of control even when they may be inappropriate (such as endangering safety by rushing into a burning building) or irrational (trying to resuscitate a dead baby). Maddi and

Kobasa, (1984) define control as a sense of autonomy and an ability to influence destiny.

2. *Cohesion:* utilizing natural or forming new support system connections to utilize social supports as a coping strategy. This means fostering propinquity beyond the artificial grouping of the debrief. The organization would do well to coordinate opportunities for naturally forming disaster work groups to have contact in a manner which facilitates informal communication and expressions of support. Frequently, the demands of the disaster, bringing workers together for the short duration of the disaster effort, results in disbursement back to regular duty assignment, shift or job rotation, or release time that further hampers informal contact. At Lockerbie, the two hour drive in small autos back to Glasgow each might due to hotel room hostages did more to facilitate debriefing than the formal debrief.

3. *Communication:* accepting and acting upon the need to talk about the event to a significant support figure(s). While those who confide their traumatic experience to someone quickly after a traumatic event that those who confide later, it is the response of the confidant that is associated with positive outcome, not the telling of the story itself. What happens between traumatized and counselor, within the group, or in the case of disaster workers, within the organization that tends to determine the success of the intervention or debrief. (Aldwin, 1994). Thus organizational and occupational cultural responses to the trauma story are as, if not more, important to worker health and restoration to duty.

4. *Challenge:* seeing the hardship and loss caused by the event as something to be overcome using one's skills, knowledge and intelligence. Maddi and Kobasa (1984) define challenge in which perceived changes can be viewed as opportunities for growth and development rather than as threats to security or survival. Even failure can be seen to produce positive results. It is important that the organization and co-workers focus on what went right or how the future will be better than to dwell on errors or identifying scapegoats.

5. *Commitment:* Remaining active in the process of resolving traumatic sequelae, including seeing a sense of meaning related to the future in regard to the experience. Maddi and Kobasa (1984) define the attribute as a sense of meaning and purpose in one's existence encompassing self, others and work.

The following components should be added to Kobasa's list:

6. *Connection:* becoming an expert on connecting reactions to trauma and following through on coping and treatment strategies and developing a schema, individual and organizational, on the meaning of the event.

7. *Clarification:* making the event understandable by gaining sufficient information to process the disaster so that freedom from confusion results.

This is especially important for individuals who utilize informative control (Taylor and Fraser, 1984) as a coping mechanism to alleviate traumatic stress. In this style, the disaster worker actively acquires factual information about the disaster and recovery. Information will be eagerly sought and persons exhibiting this type of control usually look to any official representative to supple the answers.

8. *Coherence:* making the trauma or disaster account from the reports of others into a logical and consistent story. Sullivan (1993) defines coherence as having three components: meaningfulness, comprehensibility and manageability. Antonovsky's (1987-93) concept of coherence fits well with the idea of a "healing theory" (Figley, 1989) and "meaning" (Herman, 1992) orientation of trauma resolution put forward by others.

9. *Cognition:* processing the knowing of the disaster, including the components of awareness and judgment.

10. *Commemoration:* pursuing an action to call the event to remembrance to serve as a memorial, or to make a ceremony honoring those involved in the disaster. Every individual and organization has rituals of memorial, healing and closure which need to occur.

11. *Comfort:* developing a feeling of relief or encouragement and finding a way to receive consolation in this time of trouble and worry.

12. *Closure:* to achieve a state of feeling that the disaster has ended and although the person will never be the same as before the event, that some normalcy has been retained or returned.

It is not surprising that many employee assistance program (EAP) trauma counselors have increased their efforts following workplace violence and disaster in providing consultation similar to that offered by organizational psychologists. Motivational research and theory has increasingly turned away from supervisory practices directed at individual employees, finding actions that manipulate organizational culture much more effective in having an impact on performance and productivity. EAP trauma counselors found greater promise in assisting the employer to effectively supervise the organizational culture in order to inculcate the wellness 'C's and maximize the prevention and recovery from the acute stress caused by disaster mitigation. The trauma counselor can assist the organization as well as individual disaster workers to explore and perform the tasks represented by the twelve wellness 'C's. Organizations are made up of social worlds where people talk, co-act, interact and transact with each other. Understanding the manifestations, values, beliefs and deeply-held assumptions that define organizational culture is critical to assisting work groups and their component members to master trauma.

DISASTER MENTAL HEALTH RESPONSES IN GROUPS

For economy and efficiency, group responses to major traumas involving many potentially traumatized persons are often chosen by mental health providers (Dunning, 1985, 1988). Groups provide a mechanism for responding to the needs of a large number of people as quickly and as thoroughly as possible. In work settings, group responses can provide the least disruptive way in which to address the needs of workers. It is important, however, to assess if the group approach is the best protocol to use after a traumatic event. The disaster worker may be experiencing a wide range of disturbing reactions to the event and its aftermath. Because it is true that we generally prefer to talk about upsetting and embarrassing reactions with those who are familiar to us rather than strangers, to disclose upsetting feelings in a group at this point may be even more stressful than holding them in. Herman (1992) notes that although the worker may feel comforted by the notion that he or she is not alone in the experience, in practice some workers may feel overwhelmed by a group. Hearing the details of the experience of others may prove even more disturbing or reinforce beliefs such as "See, I told you it wasn't safe out there." Figley's (1989) five-phase approach to treating traumatized families may prove a useful guide for implementing cohesive (e.g., work unit) group counseling.

It has become increasingly common, though, for group debriefings to be offered after large-scale accidents, natural disasters or crimes involving groups of people. In these types of situations, identification with fellow workers may result in the natural formation of group camaraderie among those who survived, took part in disaster response, or were identified as part of a "group" by the media. This shared identity can be an important resource for recovery, or it can result in exacerbating the fears of the worker of being identified as a victim of the event, of being vulnerable by association, or being marked by a label of invisible injury. A large group meeting for educational debriefing can facilitate preventive education concerning the consequences of the trauma, coping strategies, and resources available for resolution. If no resources currently exist, the group can act to mobilize the provision of needed services.

A group meeting immediately subsequent to a traumatic event can provide an opportunity for exchanging information on acute stress and traumatic stress reactions, identifying common symptom patterns and explaining strategies for coping and management of symptoms. The group leader must avoid creating a situation that might flood workers with overwhelming memories or feelings, engendering in them a despairing belief that the worst is not over yet. In addition, comments in group meetings run the risk of tainting the memory of those who might be called upon to testify in a legal proceeding by contaminating their recall through contact with the group.

The use of trauma counselors in acute and traumatic stress situations can be highly effective in relieving the physical, behavioral and psychological dysfunction caused by the event. The goal of such intervention is to reconstitute everyday coping behaviors and facilitate recovery for those affected by the event. Experience has shown that, although most people resolve traumatic reactions and distress on their own in a short period of time, the early provision of assessment and support services can ameliorate the deleterious sequelae in some individuals. A crucial element of acute disaster response is helping workers marshal their support systems. These resources support workers and help restore wellness by supplying physiological, psychological and social assistance.

One immediate benefit of trauma counseling conducted in the acute stage is to establish a liaison between the worker, the support system and resources that might be used to deal with sequelae that are disrupting or disturbing or are delayed for some time. Any preprinted information should provide for a variety of resources and should not be used to promote and market just one. People vary in being able to recognize their own needs and printed materials allow greater dissemination of information on resources, especially to others in the support system.

It is important that the workers believe that seeking assistance and support is in their control and that the counseling service provided is not just an attempt to expand a client base or for the employer to collect information. It is possible that some mental health professionals may take umbrage at this idea. But the reality is that the workers may reject the information, and assistance provided by mental health agencies, based on their belief that the counseling is for the benefit of the care provider or employer and not the worker, e.g., to make money, fill beds or negate the liability of the employer, which will not facilitate acceptance of necessary mental health services.

The team of trauma counselors must be aware of participants' feelings of being overwhelmed. Knowledge of the event and the workers' role during the disaster is very important. In the work setting, usually the managers of the employees involved in the event are a very good source for information. It is not advisable to include, in a group setting, different levels of employees (e.g., employees and managers). Nor should the group include the person(s) who may be blamed for a particular event, (e.g., the heavy machinery operator who was operating the machine during a rescue attempt that caused the death or injury to a survivor).

One important caution about group debriefings is that any service related to emotional and potentially litigious issues must take into account the participant's needs for psychological safety as well as legal and institutional concerns. Herman (1992) notes that just as one should never assume that a traumatized individual's family will be supportive, it is never safe to assume that a group of people who work together will be supportive of one another or develop cohesion just because they have experienced the same traumatic event. Underlying conflicts of interest may be exacerbated by the disclosure called for in the group setting. Group intervention goals in the acute stage of trauma should, therefore, focus on safety and education. The outcome of the group meeting should be primarily educational, unless the group has developed a level of trust, cohesion and support that would allow a more intense psychological approach to treating the trauma.

If the debriefing is to occur during the response period then the group should be oriented to cognitive issues rather then explorative and assessment concerns. Persons still involved in rescue operations, for example, may still need a level of denial in order to cope with their continued activities. It would be counterproductive to strip away participants' survival coping mechanisms at a time when they need them most. The group meeting should be primarily educational until the event is over. In the post-event phase, if the group has developed a level of trust, cohesion and support, then a more psychological approach could be appropriate.

CONCLUSION

In order to facilitate integration and recovery, if necessary, in disaster workers who are acutely stressed or traumatized by the event, as well as provide support to those disaster workers feeling generally stressful reactions to their assignment, it is necessary that disaster workers:

- Hear a consistent message in the context of the organization and their occupation that a variety of reactions including symptoms of anxiety, sleep disturbance, hyper-arousal, depression and so forth, are normal and are not indicative of illness or professional incompetence.
- Receive strong and explicit encouragement to resume normal personal and professional activities. Positive coping strategies related to physical well-being and the twelve C's should be stressed.
- Share the disaster experience through some method of communication (verbal or written) with a supportive listener.
- Identify and connect with social support resources.
- Be provided with opportunities and resources to develop an organizational culture which fosters hardiness and resiliency.

The work will teach you how to do it.

Estonian Proverb

DIDACTIC-EXPERIENTIAL GROUP TRAINING

Meliné Karakashian, PhD
Richard Mercer, PhD

In this section the authors present a model of counselor training and debriefing, and issues relevant to the psychological effects of crisis intervention on crisis counselors. The group of counselors were victims of the catastrophic earthquake in Soviet Armenia of December 1988. This study attempted to determine both the degree of PTSD and depression among counselors who were primary victims of the disaster and who worked with traumatized children, and also the effects of a didactic-experiential group process on the reported PTSD and depression symptoms of these counselors. Therapeutic effects of the didactic-experiential group, implications for counselor training in crisis intervention and for future research are discussed.

The field of mental health in disaster relief has grown in the past decade, with considerable attention given to crisis intervention training and debriefing of counselors (Armstrong et al., 1991; Cohen, 1992; Talbot et al., 1992). It is widely recognized among mental health professionals that trauma work affects the clinician (Alexlrod et al., 1980; Danieli, 1988; Klein & Kogan, 1988; Klein-Parker, 1988; Pines 1986). The literature indicates a scarcity of information on the effects of trauma work on counselors who themselves were victims of the trauma, and who were not privileged to receive debriefing.

A study was conducted in the course of a lecturing assignment in the earthquake ravaged city of Gumri (formerly Leninakan) in the newly independent state of Armenia. The study attempted to determine the usefulness of a didactic-experiential group counseling training program in addressing the effects of trauma work on counselors-in-training. The counselors provided psychological crisis intervention to traumatized children and consultation to parents. The first author was particularly interested in determining the prevalence of Post-traumatic stress disorder and depression symptoms in this group of counselors who were immediate victims of the disaster and the possible effects of the didactic-experiential program on these symptoms.

185

Methodology

Subjects

The participants consisted of twenty-five (25) female school counselors who lived and worked in the city of Gumri. The counselors had all experienced the horror of the earthquake and continued to live and work in the city. Of the 25, twelve (12) had lost their homes and eight (8) presently lived in temporary shelters, which had become their permanent homes since their hope of regaining a residence had vanished. At the time of the study, the Armenian autonomous enclave, Nagorno-Karabagh in neighboring Azerbaijan, was leading a struggle for independence. The latter had blockaded Armenia, preventing foodstuffs, staples and fuel from reaching the country. The study participants, already subjected to the traumatic effects of the earthquake, continued to be threatened by war and blockade.

Of the 25 subjects, 40% (ten) were at work and 40% (ten) were at home during the earthquake. They all worked as teachers at the time: 84% (twenty one) were in the company of others during the disaster; 16% (four) were physically injured requiring hospitalization; 12% (three) lost close and extended family members; 16% (four) were sole supporters of their households; 92% (twenty three) had one or more children; 92% (twenty three) were married; and 12% (three) were widowed by the disaster. This mean age was 40 and the range was 30 to 53. All 25 were born in Armenia, while their parents were survivors of the 1915-18 Genocide (Hovannisian, 1969; Sarafian, 1994).

All 25 participants worked in kindergarten and elementary schools as counselors after the earthquake. They were all certified teachers who had taken courses in pedagogy and educational psychology. They had expressed interest in becoming counselors following the earthquake and participated in a semester's coursework in "School Psychology" offered by the Teachers' Retraining Institute in Leninakan between September of 1990 and May of 1991. Most of the instructors lacked clinical expertise or knowledge of Post-traumatic Stress Disorder. Six of the 25 had also participated in two two-week seminars offered by an American psychiatrist, Edmund Gergerian and the primary author of this study, M. Karakashian in 1991. The seminars were planned pursuant to an agreement between Armen Goenjian, MD, Director of Psychiatric Outreach of the Armenian Relief Society of Western United Stares and the Ministry of Education of Armenia. The 25 participants were referred to the first author by their boards of education to participate in an intensive seminar on group therapy methods. This was, therefore, an unusual group of counselors whose professional training was elementary by American standards.

Instruments

Demographic data was gathered through a questionnaire filled in by the participants. An adaptation of the Hamilton Rating Scale for Depression (1967) was used to assess the level of depression. The adaptation consisted of presenting the key terms used by Hamilton in question format in Armenian, for clarity of understanding. This is a 17-item list of symptoms marked for severity (zero to four). The scale produces a depression score ranging from a minimum of 0 to a maximum of 68 (Hamilton, 1967). The Hamilton depression symptoms have high agreement with DSM III-R criteria for Major Depression. It is used with patients presenting both reactive and endogenous depressions (Hamilton, 1967). Reliability coefficients are reported by the author to be in the range of .84 to .90. Hamilton (1960) considered the scale to be of "practical value in assessing results of treatment." Given the intervention model of the present study, the Hamilton scale was deemed appropriate for use.

An adaptation of the Self-Report of PTSD measure (Applebaum, 1989) was used to assess Post-traumatic stress disorder symptoms in this group of counselors. It is a 17-item structured interview schedule, which inquires about DSM III-R symptoms of PTSD in a Likert format, ranging from zero to four, the latter indicating most severity. The scale measures the three diagnostic symptom clusters for PTSD, namely, Re-experiencing, Avoidance and Arousal. "According to the DSM-III-R criteria, PTSD diagnosis is reached by meeting the following DSM III-R criteria: 1 symptom for re-experiencing, 3 symptoms for Avoidance and 2 symptoms for Arousal. The Likert format allowed the assessment of the degree of disturbance reported by the respondents."

Procedure

The didactic group meetings were held in a classroom of a local school building accessible to all participants. The training sessions were held daily for three hours on seven consecutive days. The didactic-experiential group training progressed as follows.

First Meeting:

Introductory Phase: The training program was presented to the participants as a combination of lecture and direct experience in group process. The lecturer then related her interest in studying the effects of treatment of trauma on counselors who experienced the disaster. All of the counselor trainees agreed to participate in the study. They were told that the results of the questionnaires will be shared with them the following day in terms of majority group responses, thus maintaining individual privacy. The participants were asked to code the protocols in order to protect their privacy. The demographic questionnaire, and depression and PTSD scales were then administered.

Didactic Phase: The first lecture covered information on the psychological effects of natural disasters on victims and on difficulties encountered by clinicians in the treatment of trauma. At the end of the first lecture, the trainees were given a monograph on PTSD and group therapy intervention written by the researcher for the purpose of this lecturing assignment. They were asked to read through it for discussion the following day.

Second Meeting:

Didactic Phase: Feedback about the responses to the depression and PTSD measures was given to the trainees in general terms. Some of the counselors volunteered information about their personal experiences in the group setting. A demonstration of children's group process followed: The participants were encouraged to analyze the group dynamics in reference to the information they had read in the monograph.

Third Meeting:

Didactic Phase: A lecture was given on structured and unstructured group therapy methods. In particular, the subjects examined the Johari Window Group Counseling Model (Luft, 1966; Yalom, 1975) as a method of understanding self-awareness. "It is a four cell personality paradigm which clarifies the function of self-disclosure and feedback. It consists of each group member filling a four cell matrix based on one's self-perception and perception of another. The four cells are termed: Known to Self, Unknown to Self, Known to Others, and Unknown to Others. Yalom (1957, p. 466) considers it a cognitive aid in training groups."

Experiential Phase: The participants were then divided into two groups: kindergarten teachers and elementary grade teachers. They were asked to select two group leaders. The kindergarten teachers were asked to hold an unstructured group session for the first half of the period relating issues encountered in their work, while the lecturer supervised the elementary grade teachers in the structured group method (the Johari Window). The process was then reversed. The Johari Window provided an opportunity for group participants to understand the four aspects of a person's experience, the effect of self-disclosure and the benefits of feedback in self-understanding. In addition, the participants experienced a structured group activity and compared it to the unstructured sessions they held, thus understanding the two types of group process.

Fourth Meeting:

Didactic Phase: A list of coping strategies was distributed to group participants with instructions on teaching these strategies to school children. The strategies included suggestions to children on means of managing their fears, anxieties and depressed moods.

Experiential Phase: Unstructured group sessions continued with this primary researcher alternating supervision of the two groups.

Fifth Meeting:

Supervision: Group discussions were held on various topics related to school consultation, crisis intervention and treatment of trauma in general. Trainees were offered the opportunity to present cases and to ask questions on treatment issues.

Sixth Meeting:

The participants took an objective examination on the didactic information covered in order to receive a certificate of participation in the training program. Then they listened to two case presentations by a counselor who had been a teacher, and who had received supervised experience in crisis counseling in the local mental health clinic.

Seventh Meeting:

Post-test measures were administered and feedback was given on the overall performance of the group. During discussion of topics covered in the didactic experiential group process, participants reflected on the continued suffering of the Armenian people from the Genocide of 1915-18 (Hovannisian, 1988; Institut Für Armenische Fragen, 1987) to the earthquake to the on-going war in Karabagh and to the economic blockade. The majority related having interest in psychology for the purpose of helping children work through their traumatic stress and stated that this intervention work had become a reason for them to go on living after the disaster.

Results and Discussion:

The data was computer-analyzed using the SPSS program (1988). Internal consistency and test-retest reliability were assessed on both instruments. Interim consistency of the Hamilton Depression Scale using Cronbach's apha resulted in coefficient a=.78 for pre-test and a=.87 for post-test. Test-related reliability for the Hamilton scale was computed at r=.77. Interim consistency of the Self Report PTSD measure resulted in coefficient a=.84 for pre-test and a=.88 for post-test. Internal consistency was therefore considered acceptable.

Results of a paired t-test on the pre-and post measures of the depression scale indicated a significant difference (t=2.09, df=24, p<.001). The study participants' depression scores ranged from 6 to 72 for pre-test and from 2 to 68 for post-test. The overall depression score mean for the group was X=36.89 with SD=16.56 for pre-test and X=32.16 with SD=16.57 for post-test. Using the Bonferroni t-procedure, a series of planned comparisons on the individual items of the depression scale resulted in a significant difference in the reporting of gastrointestinal somatic symptoms (t=-2.28, df=24, p=.03).

Analysis of the responses of counselors diagnosed as meeting DSM III-R criteria for PTSD revealed a significant difference in the overall pre-and post testing (t=7.59, df=24. p=.00). The mean diagnosable score for the group was X=11.20 with SD=3.67 for pre-test and X=5.4 with SD=2.94 for post-test. A series of t-tests on individual items of the Self Report PTSD scale resulted in a significant difference in the measure of nightmares (t=2.45, df=24, p=.02).

Eighteen of the 25 counselors met the DSM III-R criteria for PTSD diagnosis (reporting symptoms of mild to severe categories) and 20 of the 25 met the DSM III-R criteria for major depression in the pre test data. Fifteen of the 25 met both the PTSD and depression criteria.

A comparison of the demographic variables and the frequency of symptoms of 15 counselors was assessed. The age range of the 15 was 30-53, similar to the total group's. Correlation between age and somatic symptoms (r=.73 and r=.62), loss of libido (r=.74), and midnight insomnia (r=.65). Age correlated significantly (r=.61) with intrusive thoughts were significant (p .05). Although significant, the correlations suggest moderate relationships between these variables in this unusual sample, and they do not infer causality. Post-earthquake location was found to correlate significantly with guilt (r=.61). Of the 15, 10 reported remaining in Leninakan following the earthquake, 2 being hospitalized and 3 being away from the city. Marital status was found to correlate with difficulty concentrating in the post-test. Of the 15 participants reporting depression and PTSD symptoms, 13 were married and 2 were widowed. The results of these demographic factors are interpreted with caution in view of the small size of subgroups.

In particular, a high proportion of counselors reported depressed mood (n=20), lack of interest in work and other activities (n=20), psychomotor agitation (n=16), somatic anxiety (n=12), and general somatic symptoms (n=13). PTSD symptoms of significance reported are: intrusive thoughts (n=13), restricted affect (n=13); irritability (n=13); amnesia of events (n=14); and a sense of foreshortened future (n=14). These findings are alarming considering the demanding nature of a counselor's role in the school, particularly in a region devastated by a natural disaster. These counselors who have had from none to minimal education in psychopatholgy and psychotherapy were expected to treat victims of trauma while themselves exhibiting similar symptoms as victims. The significant reduction of reported nightmares is interpreted conservatively given the small sample size.

The overall reduction of depression and PTSD diagnosis point to the possible healing effect of the didactic experiential group process. Indeed, Ochberg (1991) recognizes the therapeutic effect of instruction by including an educational component among his proposed techniques of Post-traumatic therapy. Description of DSM III-R symptoms and sharing of literature are such educational interventions (Ochberg, 1991). This lecturing assignment included dissemination of information on the psychological effects of trauma, on group therapy methods, on self-awareness and self-understanding, and on techniques of empowering clients. This, coupled with the experiential nature of the group process, seems to have contributed to the observed reduction in symptoms.

The increase in the reporting of gastrointestinal somatic symptoms could be interpreted in the context of somatic diagnosis and could be interpreted in the context of somatic arousal (van der Kolk and Greenberg, 1984). It can also be interpreted within the context of psychodynamic theory as a possible physiological reaction triggered by the uncovering of suppressed traumatic material. Considering the fact that this was a pilot study with a small and quite unusual sample available for training purposes, and in the absence of a control group, caution must be exercised in generalizing this finding. The moderately high correlation of age with intrusive thoughts is an interesting finding in need of exploration.

The two groups took some time to understand the concepts of the structured group method. The trainees eventually applied the method and expressed pleasure at discovering things in themselves of which they had not been aware. In the unstructured group, they presented case examples and spontaneously talked about their reactions to the trauma and its treatment. This opportunity provided the medium of self-expression in a group setting, their first such experience. It also provided a support system where group members naturally supported each other, identified with each other's experiences, or gave examples of their intervention approaches to a particular issue. The trainees looked toward the lecturer for direction and validation of their approaches.

They related feeling difficulty in their roles as school counselors and particularly expressed concern at being unable to distance themselves from trauma work, with a tendency to take problems home with them. A few related that they had taken children they were counseling home in an effort to nurture them.

The trainees' frequently reported difficulties were difficulty structuring private counseling sessions in the school building due to overcrowding, conflicts with teachers who resisted the counselors' presence in the schools and their interventions, and feelings of helplessness in addressing the immense psychological and practical needs of the children.

They asked for guidance in managing fine therapeutic issues that they routinely faced. In the absence of formal supervision, they looked for techniques they could learn and implement within the short time period in their difficult work. This was a challenge for the lecturer, who stressed the usefulness of peer group discussions in addressing treatment issues and in providing a therapeutic venting environment for the counselors.

Cultural aspects of crisis training (Cohen 1992) are an important consideration for communication and understanding. This particular group accepted the pro-bono training in return for hospitality. The trainees expressed their desire to host the lecturer by serving coffee and delicacies midway through class at every meeting. Hospitality is a characteristic of the Armenians, who are more likely to accept help if they return it with food and friendship.

While discussing their motivation and the psychological effects of trauma work on themselves, they expressed some insight about a vague relationship between the 1915-18 Genocide their parents survived and their present suffering. They referred to both as part of a pattern of victimization throughout history, adding that not only men victimized the Armenian people but even nature. They stated as a group that helping children was a raison d'être for living after the trauma. Working as counselors helped them forget their pain and gave them an opportunity to attempt to undo the damage of the earthquake and prepare the children for a better future.

Conclusion

The study of counselors who were subjected to the disaster and who treated children survivors revealed considerable symptoms of depression and PTSD meeting DSM III-R criteria. This group of trainees had no formal training, nor supervision, in crisis counseling. They were assigned to their positions by the Board of Education out of an urgent need for psychological support services in the earthquake zone and out of their courageous wish to help others. Their psychological reactions and adjustments were not previously addressed, nor, was the very difficult nature of trauma work by untrained counselors addressed.

The counselor trainees reported the healing effects of this didactic experiential group training proceed, corroborating other findings of the effectiveness of therapeutic groups in treatment of trauma (Rozinko & Dondershire, 1991; Solomon, et al., 1992). The didactic experiential group process resulted in the reduction of some depression and PTSD symptoms in the course of seven sessions. The findings are encouraging in that an instructional program contributed to the reduction of depression and PTSD symptoms. It is recommended that the study be duplicated with a larger group and a control group, and that the antecedents and implications of symptom changes be further evaluated. The implications for using group process as an instructional, debriefing and therapeutic method for crisis counselors who are primary victims of trauma are entertained.

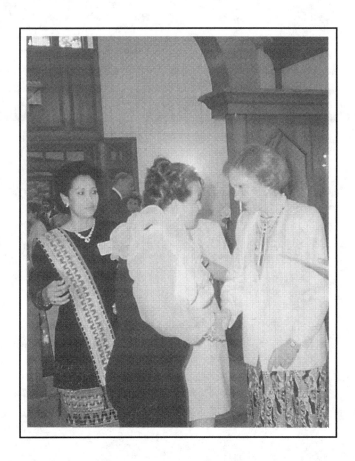

Under the patronage of the Ambassador and Mrs. M. Siregar of the Republic of Indonesia, the World Federation for Mental Health (WFMH) held an Annual Spring reception at the Siregar Mansion. The purpose of the reception was to acknowledge the dedication and achievements of scholars in the mental health field at the United Nations. Mrs. Rosalyn Carter, right, was the Honorary Chair at the reception. She congratulates Dr. Anie Sanentz Kalayjian for her involvement and achievements at the United Nations as Treasurer/Secretary of the United Nations Non-Governmental Organizations Committee on Human Rights.

May, 1994
Washington, DC

Reprinted courtesy of the *Armenian Mirror Spectator*

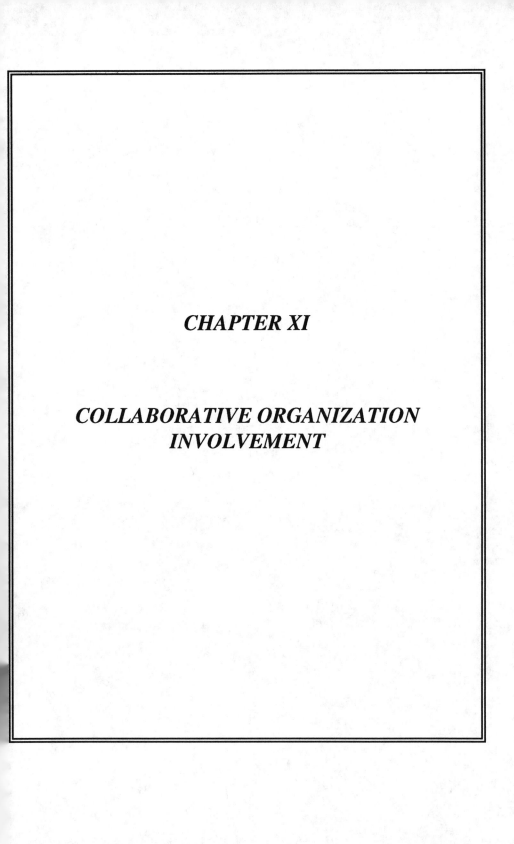

CHAPTER XI

COLLABORATIVE ORGANIZATION
INVOLVEMENT

CHAPTER XI

COLLABORATIVE ORGANIZATIONAL INVOLVEMENT

Overview

Organizational involvement is paramount primarily because the mechanisms are in place to facilitate the relief process.

This chapter highlights collaborative organizations, which are subdivided into professional, voluntary, federal, and international organizations.

The raison d'etre of a professional organization is to meet the needs of its members. Both the American Psychiatric and Psychological Associations, as well as ISTSS expressed their belief in collaboration with ARC and other agencies which oversee the relief activities. These professional organizations provided information and referrals to ARC, which has a well-established system for disaster relief.

World Federation for Mental Health (WFMH) focused on refugee trauma, be it from man-made or natural disaster. They have collaborated with the United Nations High Commissioner for Refugees (UNHCR), and the Harvard Program in Refugee Trauma (HPRT) and the Indochinese Psychiatry Clinic (IPC). After the devastating earthquake in Kobe, Japan, this group has addressed the refugee issues and proposed a plan for intervention.

The Federal Emergency Management Agency (FEMA), coordinated the national disaster relief efforts, on the Federal, state, local and volunteer and private levels. Since 1993, under the leadership of James Will, the focus of FEMA has expanded to include a comprehensive multi-hazard emergency management program as the best way to protect the nation from all hazards.

Lindy, Greene and Grace are pioneers in the study of PSTD. They consolidated forty years of trauma research and made it available to mental health professionals. The authors were most instrumental in establishing PTSD as a valid diagnosis and developed techniques for intervention.

In 1974 emotional sequelae of catastrophic events were added to the Disaster Relief Act. This provided funds for research on the psychosocial impact of disasters. Since then, the National Institute of Mental Health (NIMH) has funded a wealth of research in the field.

CARE has been providing assistance to natural disaster-ridden areas since its founding in 1945. CARE is one of the few international relief and development organizations that engages in all three phases of emergency work: disaster preparedness, response, and recovery. In all relief situations, CARE aims to move communities as quickly as possible from disaster relief to normal living conditions through long-term development.

No man is an island entire of itself.

John Donne, 1624

American Psychiatric Association (APA)

In 1992, following Hurricanes Andrew and Iniki, APA's Division of Public Affairs developed a plan for local Psychiatric Societies and other mental health providers to use in the aftermath of disasters. This plan, according to Walter S. Hill (1994), APA's Public Affairs Network Coordinator, focuses on three areas:

- Media relations,

- Referral services for the public, and

- Intervention with community leaders.

Media Relations

In 1993, The APA, in collaboration with the American Academy of Child and Adolescent Psychiatry, the National Alliance for the Mentally Ill, and the National Mental Health Association, compiled and produced a booklet entitled *Idea & Information Exchange for Disaster Response.* Media relations involves preparing press releases, a roster of expert spokespersons, and a list of mental health organizations for referrals.

Referral Services for the Public

The APA believes in collaboration with the American Red Cross and other agencies that will oversee the relief activities, rather than trying to do the outreach alone. Therefore, establishing a toll free 800-number for information and referral is important. Area hospitals can also be a good source for providing toll-free numbers, as well as appropriate staff to answer disaster-related calls.

Intervention with Community Leaders

The APA believes in making mental health professionals available for educating personnel so they may recognize the symptoms of stress-related disorders and so they know the sources of care available. Personnel referred would include teachers, clergy, physicians, social workers, elected officials, civic leaders, corporate executives, police, firefighters, hospital directors, emergency workers, insurance adjusters and others who confront the emotional crises of the disaster victims.

The readiness is all.

William Shakespeare

American Psychological Association (APA)

Durand F. Jacobs, PhD

On the occasion of its Centennial Celebration in Washington, DC in August 1992, APA presented a "Gift to the Nation" namely, a country-wide network of psychologists specially trained to provide pro bono emergency mental health services to help their neighbors when disaster strikes.

Over 300 Psychologists in California have been trained by the American Red Cross (ARC) in a 2-day course designed specifically to integrate mental health professionals as volunteers within Red Cross emergency operations. This training equipped participants with the specialized crisis intervention, counseling and debriefing skills necessary to effectively address and ameliorate Post-traumatic stress reactions among victims, helpers and their respective families and close associates.

Since pioneering this "grassroots-based" model for disaster preparedness and rapid response, these psychologists have been called out in one community or another to provide their pro bono services following mass shooting sprees, bank robberies, industrial accidents, major floods, wild fires, airplane crashes, auto pileups, toxic spills and hotel and family residence fires. Over seventy of these psychologists received individual citations from the then President of the APA for on-site services during the weeks following the Los Angeles riots in 1992. An equal number received citations from the succeeding APA President for their invaluable contributions to victims and helpers after the devastating Southern California forest fires of 1993. Over one hundred of these specially trained psychologists volunteered to support the ARC and FEMA in providing specialized services to victims and helpers after the destructive earthquake in Southern California in early 1994.

A formal Statement of Understanding has been ratified that specifies the methods of cooperation that APA and ARC and their respective state and local affiliates will exercise when preparing for and dealing with mental health needs in disaster relief situations. APA is confident that America's psychologists can mobilize for community service just as 10,000 volunteered to provide free mental health assistance to victims and their families during the Persian Gulf War.

The following Interim Project Report is titled, "Suggestions to State Psychiatric Associations (SPA's) for Organizing and Implementing a Disaster Response Program." It is based on experiences and observations of psychologists who have been active participants in the APA-CPA (California Psychological Association) Disaster Response Project at both state and grassroots levels.

APA-CPA Disaster Response Project

Interim Project Report

Introduction

In November 1991, the ARC released to its 2,700 local chapters a first-of-its-kind set of directives that will guide the organization and delivery of their new Disaster Mental Health Services program. These services, henceforth, will be activated whenever Red Cross assistance is requested following a catastrophe. To successfully operate this new addition to their humanitarian efforts, ARC required extensive participation of pre-trained volunteer psychologists, as well as other mental health professionals, from all over America.

In direct support of this endeavor, a formal Statement of Understanding was then ratified. It specified the methods of cooperation that APA, ARC and their respective state and local affiliates will exercise when preparing for and dealing with mental health needs in disaster relief situation.

The purpose of the Interim Report was to stimulate and assist SPA's organize and implement their individual disaster response activities. Indeed, the ultimate success of collaborative APA-ARC disaster relief planning at the national level will depend entirely on the extent of effective networking accomplished at the "grassroots" level by their respective state and local affiliates.

In March of 1991 an Initial Project Report was distributed to all SPA presidents. The report described how CPA had mobilized resources of its central office and affiliated chapters to create a disaster response program, how liaison was established with the California ARC and the California Department of Mental Health (DMH) at both state and local levels, and how increasing numbers of CPA members had joined local Disaster Response Committees in each of its 23 chapters and were taking the Red Cross 2-day "Crisis Intervention in Disaster" course designed for mental health professionals. Completion of this training is a prerequisite for California psychologists to become volunteer members of local Red Cross Crisis Intervention Teams.

During 1991, many of these psychologists responded to Red Cross calls for assistance in single-family home fires, a hotel fire, a toxic spill, an earthquake in Pasadena, a multiple airplane crash at the Los Angeles Airport, and the firestorm in Oakland, California.

At the end of the Project, a full description of CPA's experiences, accumulated resource materials, and recommendations for SPAs interested in pursuing similar disaster response activities will be compiled in a Workbook/Procedures Manual.

"A Gift to the Nation" included the following:

I. How to Build a Disaster Response Capability

- Recognize that APA has encouraged your Association to take a critical role in implementing the Statement of Understanding (SOU) now in effect between APA and the ARC.
- While referencing the SOU, produce a mission statement to guide activities of an appropriately named disaster response committee.
- Appoint a qualified and energetic chair who can devote the considerable time needed to establish and maintain liaison with state and local level ARC and DMH representative.
- Involve your leadership (i.e., officers, board of directs and other highly visible members) in this activity as role models and as analytic agents.
- Keep your disaster response program highly visible and relevant to your general membership.
- Plan a series of articles in your newsletter on Post-traumatic stress, vulnerability of children and elders to emotional trauma, treating reactions to critical incidents such as rage, the unexpected death of a teacher or a fellow worker, and a series of adolescent suicides. The objective is to impress upon your members that disaster-related training is directly applicable to their day-to-day practice. This approach will help overcome the resistance of busy private practitioners to give the time required for Red Cross training and related drills.
- Make disaster response plans and activities an agenda item at all board and chapter meetings. Emphasize both the intrinsic and extrinsic benefits of highly visible public service participation by psychologists at the local community level. Don't be shy about indicating that this can be an excellent marketing vehicle.
- It is important that your Association's disaster committee chairperson remain in close and continuing telephone contact with local chapter or regional meetings to aid in recruitment, reinforce exceptional achievements,

- participate in community disaster planning meetings and otherwise provide direct support to the efforts of the local disaster committee.
- Keep the system simple and self-sustaining at both the state and local level. Try to maintain continuity of both state and local disaster committee chairs to avoid stop and start problems.
- The major emphasis should be focused on grassroots networking between local psychologists and the local ARC chapter, as well as any additional local agencies they choose to support.
- The state association's role should be to provide information and support and to network with state-level agencies as needed.
- While your first commitment will be to provide emergency support to local ARC chapters and mental health agencies, also encourage ARC trained psychologists to network with other community groups of their own choosing. Let each group know that local psychologists stand ready to help their neighbors when disaster strikes.
- Establish a "lending library" in your Association's central office. Collect and distribute disaster-related materials to your chapters and other interested members. Provide an annotated bibliography of disaster related references and a list of free brochures available from the Emergency Services Branch of the National Institute of Mental Health.
- SPAs should consider restricting member participation in disaster response activities to licensed psychologists who, among other considerations, are subject to state statutory controls and also to following the principles of their Association's ethical code when providing professional services of any kind.
- At the outset expect a very uneven reception to your disaster response program among chapters and members. They may be already committed to other pro bono activities. However, marketing this program as part of a highly visible country-wide enterprise between the ARC and APA and their respective state and local affiliates can only help.
- Before disaster strikes, participating psychologists might seek to establish channels of communication with "gate keepers" of the differing ethnic groups in and around their community (e.g., Hispanic, Asian, Native American). Through these trusted intermediaries, psychologists may serve in a consultative or direct fashion when extending services to persons whose cultural background and language may be different from their own.
- Disasters don't respect normal working hours. The California experience has underscored the importance of having readily available to your disaster committee chair and others with a need to know names, addresses and both office and home telephone numbers of psychologists involved in the disaster response program. If your resources permit, keep this information current in a computer file at Association headquarters.

- When you can, upgrade this basic information on each participating psychologist with languages spoken and notations on their disaster-relevant clinical experience (e.g., with children, serious mentally ill, substance abusers). Also, with permission, distribute current copies of this listing to appropriate ARC and DMH officials with whom you are collaborating. They may need to have this information at hand to overcome communication breakdowns in a major disaster.
- Since the ARC does not respond to all disasters, you might wish to consider making contact with your state/provincial DMH. Let them know about the availability of psychologists who have been trained as ARC volunteers to provide emergency mental health services in the event of a disaster.
- Don't be surprised or upset to learn that "Disaster Preparedness Plans" of most states and large municipalities do not recognize or include means for dealing with repercussions of the psychological impact of disaster upon victims, helpers and their families. Since the ARC does not respond to all catastrophes that may impact a community, SPA's may wish to offer consultation to these governmental groups about the importance of incorporating psychological services in their disaster plans.
- Inform the media how psychologists in your state/province have prepared themselves through specialized training to provide free services to their neighbors when disaster strikes. When doing so, provide names and photos of local psychologists so that their home community is made aware of their pro bono activities.
- Your Governmental Affairs Committee might also keep legislative representatives appraised of this commendable pro bono activity by local psychologists to assist constituents in their districts.

II. Networking with the ARC and Other Agencies at the State and Grassroots Levels.

- All ARC chapters and SPA's were sent a copy of the SOU between the ARC and APA. This spells out the cooperative relationships now in force between these two organizations and their respective state and local affiliates for anticipating and dealing with mental health needs when disaster strikes.
- The availability of these two documents will facilitate prompt networking between members of SPAs and their state and local ARC representatives and assure them that members of your Association stand ready to join with them to implement the objectives set forth in the aforementioned documents.

- The California experience has shown that you can rapidly assemble relatively large numbers of psychologists to be trained by, and then become affiliated with, ARC chapters located in the larger metropolitan areas. When disasters have occurred in more remote or thinly populated area, these larger chapters have responded to requests by smaller chapters to send a Crisis Intervention Team to the stricken community.

- Even when local psychologists are available as members of ARC Crisis Intervention Teams in thinly populated areas, their numbers are usually quite modest, and burnout occurs very rapidly. In these instances, the larger chapters may be called upon when local resources are exhausted. Moreover, psychologists from communities not in the disaster area can be utilized in the debriefing of psychologists and other helpers who have been directly involved at the disaster scene.

- Be aware that, historically, most local ARC chapters have not been particularly sensitive to the need for providing psychological assistance to disaster victims or to their own overworked staff and volunteers. The smaller chapters also will be hard-pressed to add a "disaster mental health services" component to their current duties. Consequently, you can anticipate that in most cases offers of assistance by local psychologists to staff or even to head their Crisis Intervention Teams will be warmly received.

- Until sufficient numbers of local psychologists have an opportunity to take the official ARC disaster mental health course, it may be helpful to consult with leaders of local chapters about the possibility of "grandparenting" local psychologists who can document equivalent training, providing they also complete basic orientation to ARC disaster procedures. Grandparenting may prove to be an effective means of quickly gathering enough trained psychologists to constitute a Crisis Intervention Team, while requiring that later applicants must complete the official ARC course as it becomes available.

- In California, we have found that one way to maintain the interest of psychologists certified members of ARC Crisis Intervention Team is to have them called out occasionally to assist victims of single family home fires that occur all too frequently in their own community. This helps strengthen their crisis intervention skills and encourages them to remain active in the program.

- Another way to maintain interest is to encourage certified psychologists to participate in periodic ARC disaster drills or in drills organized by the county or state office of Emergency Services.

PROFESSIONAL ETHICAL AND LEGAL ISSUES

The psychologist's role in providing emergency disaster relief services is best described as educational and supportive and performed within a limited time frame. In the types of crisis counseling and debriefing activities that transpire in a disaster context, a formal therapeutic relationship or contract is not established.

The CPA Ethics Committee Chair has suggested the following approach with victims and/or helpers: "This is probably the only time I will see you. But, I'm here to help you as much as I can now." When indicated, give victims or helpers written information regarding how to get back to the ARC or local mental health department should they require further psychological assistance in the future. It is considered unprofessional to distribute personal business cards to victims, helpers or their families under disaster conditions.

All immediate post-disaster victims and helpers or their families are entitled to the same constraints on confidentiality as are operative in professional practice. This is especially important to note when dealing with the media. When functioning under direct ARC or DMH auspices at a disaster scene, it is wise to refer all media inquiries or interview invitations to the designated media contact person of the supervising agency.

To be a man means
to be a fellow man.

Leo Laeck

Cooperative for Assistance and Relief Everywhere (CARE)

Elizabeth Puckett, BA

CARE has been helping victims of natural disasters since its founding in 1945. CARE is one of the few international relief and development organizations that engages in all three phases of emergency work. These three phases include:

1. Disaster preparedness and prevention,
2. Disaster response, and
3. Disaster recovery.

CARE employs a variety of methods in addressing these three phases of emergency work. The Emergency and Assistance Unit (EAU) at CARE-USA headquarters coordinates and provides guidance in emergency work to CARE's missions worldwide. Individual country missions develop their own disaster plans and incorporate them into their regular operating plans. CARE designs and installs disaster warning systems in conjunction with other relief organizations. Tree planting is taught and employed as a preventative measure for landslide and flood control. Food, water, water purification tablets, vehicles and material for constructing shelters are pre-positioned for natural disaster preparedness.

An example of disaster preparedness and prevention can be seen at CARE-Nepal's Bengas Tal/Rupa Tal and Syangja Watershed Management project. This project helps hundreds of farm families increase food production. The techniques used also help to conserve topsoil and prevent flooding and landslides.

CARE bases its ability to respond quickly and effectively to disasters on mobilizing and coordinating available resources. In 1993, CARE provided food, medicine, temporary shelter and tools to more than 11 million victims of catastrophic disasters worldwide.

In all relief situations, CARE aims to move as quickly as possible from disaster relief to normal living conditions through long-term development. For example, in CARE-Ethiopia's Shoa Rehabilitation Project, CARE operated a food for work program. This project provides food for 60,000 people in return for their work on drought recovery activities such as hillside terracing, road construction and rehabilitation, tree planting and irrigation. CARE is working with communities to help restore the agricultural base and improve the nutritional status in the region.

CARE evaluates and monitors all of its projects on a regular basis. We compare data collected prior to, during and after a project to measure its accomplishments. Through monitoring, CARE ensures that all systems are functioning properly and having the desired effect.

I am still learning.

Michaelangelo's Motto

Federal Emergency Management Agency (FEMA)

James L. Will, FEMA Director

MISSION STATEMENT

This mission of FEMA is to provide the leadership and support to reduce the loss of life and property and protect our institutions from all types of hazards through a comprehensive, risk-based, all-hazards emergency management program of mitigation, preparedness, response and recovery.

We have a unique opportunity as a nation (and at FEMA) to develop an effective and efficient nationwide emergency management system that will significantly reduce the impact of disasters on victims and our communities and also reduce the costs, to all parties, of responding to and recovering from such disasters.

FEMA's mission stresses that FEMA has a leadership, coordination and management role that focuses on reducing risks and helping victims of disasters, regardless of the cause. This role applies to federal agencies, state and local governments and private and volunteer organizations involved in disaster relief, as well as to disaster victims who receive assistance directly from the federal government.

This mission denotes that FEMA's leadership and support will focus on the most likely risks, such as hurricanes, earthquakes or floods, that a jurisdiction faces. Through developing the capability to respond to specific risks, emergency management capabilities will exist for any hazard.

FEMA's GOALS

To accomplish FEMA's mission, the following goals shape the priorities and policies to be implemented:
- To create an emergency management partnership with other Federal agencies, State and local governments, volunteer organizations and the private sector;

- To establish, in concert with FEMA's partners, a national emergency management system that is comprehensive, risk-based and all-hazards in approach;
- To make hazard mitigation the foundation of the national emergency management system;
- To provide a rapid and effective response to any disaster; and,
- To strengthen state and local emergency management.

To implement these priorities FEMA has adopted the following policies and taken the following actions since I became FEMA Director in April 1993.

Establish a New Emergency Management Partnership

FEMA is developing a new partnership in providing emergency management services. This is a program wherein state (hereafter this term includes the District of Columbia and Caribbean and Pacific Island Territories) and local emergency management agencies, and private organizations are partners in planning and executing their emergency management responsibilities.

In this way, the ideas and concerns of all parties can be incorporated into the process, and response and recovery activities can be effectively coordinated through planning and exercises based upon ongoing cooperative relationships.

FEMA has initiated a number of activities in order to make this goal a reality. FEMA has prepared a draft Interstate Compact, and has encouraged the states and territories to adopt it, or a revised version, as a mutual aid agreement. Currently, 34 states have adopted such a compact or included mutual aid in their executive legislation.

FEMA has also prepared agreements that define how FEMA will work with the states in the event of a major disaster. As of August 1994, almost all the states have signed mutual aid agreements with FEMA. These agreements define how FEMA will work together with the states on major events — especially during the initial period after the prediction or occurrence of a disaster.

I have reduced the administrative load on State and local agencies receiving FEMA funds. These changes were made effective for the Fiscal Year 1994 Comprehensive Cooperative Agreement (CCA) negotiations. CCA's are the mechanism used by FEMA to provide financial assistance to states for emergency management activities.

FEMA gave the states, in the FY 1994 CCA, the flexibility to develop their own priorities and corresponding programs so that they could accomplish risk-based assessments without undue restrictions from FEMA.

The requirements are now performance-based and focus on program accomplishments. In FY 1995, there will be even more changes as FEMA plans to use functional rather than programmatic annexes.

For example, all of the planning requirements will be incorporated into one section, all exercise requirements in another section, and so forth.

As a general practice, FEMA Headquarters and Regional personnel have been asked to spend as much time as possible working with state and local organizations. This practice will enable FEMA personnel to become better acquainted with their counterparts at the state and local level, and to better understand the emergency management organizations, policies and procedures used by these agencies. It will also lead to the kind of teamwork that needs to be in place at a disaster scene.

In addition, FEMA Regional Directors have assigned an employee to work with the Governor and emergency management director at the State Emergency Operations Center immediately upon occurrence of a disaster warning or event.

Manage by Means of an All-hazards Approach

When I became Director of FEMA, I proposed that FEMA adopt an all-hazards emergency management program, which covers natural and technological hazards and even prepares for what is hopefully the remote possibility of foreign attack.

There has been much discussion concerning whether FEMA's program should be civil defense or a multi-hazard emergency management program. There are those who have said these functions must be separate, that is FEMA should administer a program for foreign attack that is separate from one which prepares the nation for natural and technological hazards.

I disagree. I believe that a multi-hazard program with provision for factors unique to certain types of emergencies is the most cost-effective way to prepare for all emergencies, and especially, it is the best way to protect the Nation from all hazards. The best civil defense capability is achieved through a comprehensive multi-hazard emergency management program.

Disasters are stressful situations, and under stress people tend to revert to first-learned behavior. Day-to-day response, recovery and reconstruction activities are handled on a regular basis for natural and technological hazards.

If a foreign attack does occur, it is very important that as many as possible of these same procedures be used rather than using a separate plan with separate procedures, expecting disaster personnel to switch to those procedures in the midst of a catastrophe.

FEMA has adopted the all-hazard concept and we have suggested that state and local emergency management agencies do the same. Programs within FEMA now conduct their activities based upon the all-hazard concept.

Establish Mitigation as the Foundation of Emergency Management

FEMA's primary mission is first to do everything reasonably possible to mitigate the effects of a disaster, that is, to prevent injuries, deaths, property damage and economic losses, and to minimize where they cannot be prevented.

Many aspects of disaster mitigation can be conducted with relatively little expenditure of time and money. At the very least, we must stop building structures which could be dangerous to occupants during a disaster. This can be accomplished by:

1. Not building in dangerous areas, such as flood zones or earthquake areas subject to soil liquefaction;
2. Ensuring that all buildings are constructed according to one of the current national building codes and other applicable standards; and,
3. Modifying existing structures by anchoring buildings to their foundations, and securing furnishings so they cannot fall on occupants or block exits.

Every new structure which is correctly located and built to code, or modified, is one less building we have to worry about in the future. Then, in 20 years, for example, a good percentage of the buildings in use would have built-in mitigation, resulting in significant progress in reducing disaster-caused human suffering and the corresponding costs of providing assistance.

FEMA's national mitigation goal is, by the year 2020, to engender a fundamental change in public attitude which demands safer communities in which to live and work and, thereby, to reduce by at least half, the loss of life, injuries, economic costs and destruction of natural and cultural resources which result from the occurrence of natural disaster.

In order to implement mitigation actions on a national scale, FEMA has created, for the first time ever, a Mitigation Directorate, which is developing a comprehensive national mitigation strategy with our Federal agency partners, the Congress, state and local governments, academia, the private sector and individual citizens. We are also organizing an interagency task force among our Federal partners to draft a Federal mitigation plan for pre- and post-disaster Federal leadership and coordination, much in the same way that the Federal Response Plan establishes a framework for disaster response efforts.

The cornerstone of our strategy must be the acceptance by all Americans of the need to take personal responsibility for making their community a safe place to live and prosper. Government and the private sector must provide leadership, coordination and research support including real financial incentives that support communities, businesses and individuals who undertake mitigation actions.

The National Mitigation Strategy will offer innovative approaches for combining funds and coordinating public efforts with the private sector and, indeed, with every American. It will offer an opportunity for each of our citizens, and for their communities, to invest in themselves and in the future.

The ultimate success of the strategy is based on the critical need for all Americans to support mitigation in their communities. Communities must demand that contractors build stronger buildings and realtors disclose any known hazards to prospective buyers, and that local officials enforce building codes, zoning and environmental laws for everyone.

FEMA has also built mitigation into other program areas. For example, for the first time ever, a senior FEMA official whose sole responsibility was to identify and investigate mitigation opportunities was assigned to the response and recovery efforts for the 1994 Northridge Earthquake. Additionally, FEMA provided financial assistance to the State of California in accordance with the state's mitigation plan that had been prepared prior to the earthquake. FEMA is promoting the California example of pre-planning mitigation activities with other states around the country.

Pro-active, pre-disaster mitigation measures aggressively pursued and supported through innovative incentives can reduce disaster assistance costs. For example, FEMA's Midwest Buyout Program recently committed to spending over $76 million over the next five years in the 40 Missouri communities to relocate homes, businesses and, in some cases, entire communities out of the flood-plain. It is estimated that these actions will save over $200 million in losses in the next 15 years. As of August 1994, over 7,100 parcels of land in the nine midwest states have been approved for purchase, thereby moving thousands of individuals and businesses out of harm's way.

Develop a Strong Disaster Response and Recovery Capability

It is not possible for FEMA to establish a comprehensive emergency management program without involvement in the response phase, because, even with formal notification to all parties and announcements to the public that this is not part of the agency's mission, when a disaster occurs the general expectation is the FEMA will respond immediately. Therefore, I believe the only option is to recognize the perceptions and expectations and develop a program incorporating a response role for FEMA.

Of course, FEMA can never be a "first responder" agency, as that is the function of local and state governments. However, FEMA is addressing the issue of participation in the response phase of a disaster in cooperation with state and local emergency management directors, and is developing a comprehensive coordinated program which meets the needs of the state and local governments in protecting our citizens.

One component of this effort is the development and refinement of the Federal Response Plan (FRP). The FRP provides the operational and planning framework for the coordination by FEMA of Federal government's efforts in a disaster response and recovery operation. Twenty-eight Federal departments and agencies along with the ARC participate in the FRP. The FRP was employed formally for the first time during the Northridge Earthquake.

FEMA continues to review its options for the pre-deployment of Federal assets in anticipation of a disaster. It should be noted that any pre-deployment of Federal assets will be done in close cooperation with the states. FEMA is working with the States in developing detailed, pre-negotiated memoranda of understanding so that any pre-deployment will be made in partnership, not just unilaterally by the Federal Government.

Strengthen State and Local Emergency Management Programs

FEMA does not extinguish fires, treat victims' injuries, nor operate shelters. These services are generally provided by state and local governments and private organizations such as the ARC. Therefore, it is essential that the nation have strong emergency management programs at state and local levels.

State and local emergency management programs must have adequate resources for the risks their communities face. These programs must have sufficient personnel, qualified for their assignments, who receive frequent training and opportunities to participate in realistic exercises. A strong state and local emergency management organization reduces the need for Federal intervention.

FEMA is committed to doing everything possible to make sure that State and local emergency management agencies receive the maximum possible support. FEMA has encouraged states to consider the use of the professional standards for state and local emergency managers as a way to strengthen their capabilities.

Another way to build State and local capability is through comprehensive training programs that involve all levels of government and private agencies and organizations. And then exercise these plans and personnel at all levels. Exercises are vital to test plans to make sure that they work, and then to train personnel who will be using the plans.

However, it is important that exercises are realistic: the exercise must accurately represent the risk, and incorporate the real-world difficulties associated with disaster response and recovery. It is also important that all appropriate personnel participate in the exercises, including representatives of Federal, state, local and private organizations.

These participants must include management and administration personnel who will be involved in a disaster but rarely find the time to participate in an exercise. People who are going to work together on a disaster must first train and exercise together. The scene of a disaster is no place to meet disaster workers or read the Emergency Operations Plan (EOP).

FEMA is also emphasizing evaluation of exercises. It's never enough just to exercise without correcting problems that have been identified. We are only as good as we play — if we play poorly, then we will respond poorly. Evaluation helps us to correct those problems.

FEMA has developed an Exercise Evaluation Guide that will help State and local programs in designing evaluation programs for their exercises. FEMA implemented the new Emergency Management Exercise Reporting System in 1994 that, for the first time, allows programs to track exercises based on functions and identify areas where they are looking for corrective action.

This will also allow FEMA and its State and local partners to focus on particular problem areas in budgeting and strategic planning. People such as mayors, city managers, county commissioners and finance and purchasing officials need to be included.

CONCLUSION

During the two year period from August 24, 1992, the day Hurricane Andrew made landfall in Florida, through August 24, 1994, a period during which two of the costliest disasters in our nation's history occurred (the Midwest Floods of 1993 and the 1994 Northridge Earthquake), a total of 1,259,040 individuals applied for FEMA assistance. During this same period hundreds of American communities also applied to FEMA for aid.

America can no longer afford the disruptions to its communities and citizens nor the growing costs incurred by these disasters. FEMA is committed to working with the American people and the country's public and private institutions to reduce these costs and mitigate the negative impacts of disasters.

FEMA is also committed to forging the strongest partnerships possible with our Federal, state and local partners in emergency management to ensure that when disaster strikes, the response is quick and the recovery begins immediately.

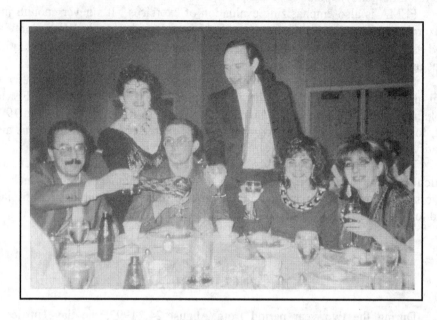

One year after the earthquake in Armenia, and two weeks after the 1989
earthquake in San Francisco: mental health professionals from Armenia
and the U.S. at the banquet of ISTSS Annual Conference, celebrating the
success of their panel discussions of their research on disasters.
San Francisco, California
October, 1989

Behind an able person
there are always other able people.

Chinese Proverb

International Society for Traumatic Stress Studies (ISTSS)

Yael Danieli, PhD

Care for disaster victims and their caregivers has been one of the major concerns of the ISTSS since its inception. Many ISTSS members are world experts in the disaster field, who, in line with the Society's mission, use all of its modes of communication and education to share their research, theoretical formulations, innovative clinical strategies and public policy concerns with colleagues around the world.

The ISTSS was established in March of 1985 to provide a forum for the sharing of related research, clinical strategies, public policy concerns and theoretical formulations in the United States and around the world. The Society is dedicated to the discovery and development of knowledge and to the stimulation of policy, program and service initiatives that seek to prevent traumatic stress and reduce its immediate and long-term consequences.

Over 1,800 mental health, social service, religious, media and legal professionals in the public and private sectors, from more than 40 countries, are currently members of the Society. Members include professionals who work with victims of all crimes and family and community violence, Holocaust and Genocide survivors, refugees, torture victims, victims of abuse, neglect, exploitation and oppression, war veterans, persons in high-risk occupations such as military, police, fire, emergency medical services or disaster workers, survivors of natural and technological disasters, persons suffering physical trauma, survivors of personal and collective tragedies, and persons committed to peace, justice development, and the protection of the environment.

Since 1985 the Society has regularly held annual, regional world, mid-year meetings in the United States, and co-sponsored meetings in both the United States and around the world. The *Journal of Traumatic Stress,* published by ISTSS since its inception, reflects both the Society's scholarly and scientific ideals and its international composition and commitment. Its international standing and contributions are also demonstrated by the adoption by the United Nations Economic and Social Council of the *Initial Report of the Society's 1989*

Presidential Task Force on Curriculum, Education and Training (E/AC.57/1990/NGO.3) as an instrument, among others (E/1990/22), of implementing the United Nations Declaration of Basic Principals of Justice for Victims of Crime and Abuse of Power (A/RES/40/34). This Report contains model curricula formulated by leading international specialists in the field and is composed of subcommittees representing different technical specialties or interests including psychiatry, psychology, social work, nursing, creative arts therapy, clergy, media, organizations, institutions and public health agencies, paraprofessionals and other professionals and undergraduate education areas. Various sections of the Report contain disaster-related materials.

The United Nations recognized the Society's contribution by granting it consultative status with the Economic and Social Council in 1993. This new role enables the Society to interface formally with United Nations activities related to disasters around the world, including those of other pertinent non-governmental organizations such as the International League of Red Cross and Red Crescent Societies. Members of the Society function as consultants to the key agencies involved in disasters, such as the United States Federal Emergency Management Agency, the National Institute of Mental Health and the Federal Bureau of Investigation and also, to the international agencies such as relevant bodies of the United Nations system.

Through its association with the United States Department of Veterans Affairs' National Center for Post-traumatic Stress Disorder, the Society provides its members with the PTSD Research Quarterly and Clinical Quarterly. In addition to its various meetings, one of the Society's main vehicles for networking and updating the work of committees and interest areas is the *Traumatic Stress Points*, the Society's Quarterly Newsletter.

The Society's commitment to disaster assistance is evidenced in the choice of keynote speakers as well as other presentations at the Society's meetings, regular reports and articles, and special issues in the publications mentioned above. Immediately after the devastating earthquake in Armenia in 1988, two of the Society's members — Drs. Kalayjian and Pynoos — were instrumental in assisting to alleviate the impact of the disaster; Dr. Kalayjian from the East Coast co-founded the Mental Health Outreach Program for Armenia, and Dr. Pynoos from the West Coast consulted and helped with data analysis.

In an ironic twist of circumstance, over 500 mental health, social service, religious and legal professionals from the US and 36 countries around the world were planning to attend the Fifth Annual Meeting of the Society for Traumatic Stress Studies in San Francisco, California, October 29 and 30, 1989. A major earthquake occurred October 17 in the San FranciscoBay Area. Society officials, sensing the prevailing feeling in the membership of "if we don't, who will?" decided to hold the meeting nevertheless, and to redirect substantial attention at various levels to the immediate and long-term needs created by Loma Prieta.

Many Society members from the area were already actively involved in the disaster relief work; many more made arrangements to arrive early from all over the world in order to assist. Some missed the scheduled professional activities in order to provide education, training, support and counseling services in the field. Efforts were undertaken to provide information via the media on the possible emotional aftershocks of natural disasters to the community, to offer special training for helping professionals, and to assist the mental health networks in providing human and clinical services to those in need.

In addition to a variety of other programs which related to the emotional recovery of persons from natural disasters as well as many other topics included in the overall program of the meeting, one of the long-planned Pre-Meeting Institutes proposed formally for Friday, October 27, was on "Post-Disaster Briefing." In its description, participants were advised that they would "travel off the hotel site to participate in a disaster drill," that "this is an experiential program where people will be asked to act as victims and participate in a debriefing," and that to wear "casual clothing and walking shoes." As Don Lattin, a reporter for the *San Francisco Chronicle* described it on October 26, "Mother Nature provided the real thing," and the workshop, re-titled Post-Earthquake Counseling" was offered, free of charge, to mental health, social service, religious and education professionals in the San FranciscoBay area. Also, on that Friday afternoon, the Society's originally scheduled opening ceremony, the "Commemoration for Victim/Survivors: A Memorial Service for Persons of All Nations, All Cultures, All Groups and All Faiths," was held in Union Square, was open to the public and also included a time of prayer for the dead and the living of San Francisco and the Bay area.

On Friday evening, October 27 at the Parc Fifty Hotel, the Society sponsored an "Open Discussion for the Community with an International Forum of Experts on Earthquake Disaster Relief" that was open to the public. Mental health experts from Australia, China, Europe, Mexico, the (then) Soviet Union and the United States shared their experiences on earthquake disaster and responded to questions from those who attended. Some participants followed Loma Prieta by doing research and presenting their findings in future Society programs and publications. Members have similarly been involved in most major disasters, albeit not in conjunction with the Society's Meetings.

Shared joy is double joy, and
Shared sorrow is half sorrow.

Swedish proverb

National Institute of Mental Health
and
Other Federal Support

Calvin J. Frederick, PhD

Major disasters have brought untold devastation upon populations world-wide since ancient times, but it is only relatively recently that the emotional and psychological effects of disaster were considered. As recently as 1976, an earthquake in Tangshan, China, killed more than 655,000 persons. The largest loss of life in modern times occurred in 1931 when floods and tidal waves from the Hunag-Ho river in China apparently took an estimated 3.7 million lives. The greatest loss of life in the US took place in 1900 in Galveston, Texas when 6,000 persons died as the result of a hurricane and flooding. Despite such devastating loss of life and property, it is only relatively recently that the psychological effects of disasters have received needed attention.

Historical Highlights of Federal Involvement

Initially attached administratively to the White House, disaster officials paid little attention to the mental and emotional sequelae of catastrophic events until passage of the Disaster Relief Act of 1974. Coincidentally, shortly thereafter, in 1979 when the Three Mile Island accident occurred, there were forty-two major presidentially declared disasters in twenty five states, Puerto Rico, the Virgin Islands and American Samoa. Disaster assistance from the Federal government exceeded $3.1 billion; yet, only $184,000 was spent for debilitating psychological disorders. Through Public Law 93-288 of the Disaster Relief Act of 1974, the Federal Disaster Assistance Administration (FDAA), now FEMA, was empowered to provide assistance to victims of disasters which exceeded the capability of local and State government to manage without outside assistance. Psychological support could be provided with the assistance of a State mental health authority and the NIMH through Section 413 of the Act. In 1976, with the assistance of FEMA personnel, it became this author's privilege to write the rules and regulations governing the provision which were published in the Federal Register. Federally authorized persons had to assess the extent of damage and recommend what was needed to restore the community to some semblance of normal functioning through building reconstruction and psychological crisis counseling. Clinics and other groups deemed competent to render appropriate services could apply for grants or contracts through the NIMH office in order to receive funding through State and Federal channels.

By recognizing the catastrophic nature of numerous unpredictable disasters annually, the US Congress committed the resources of the Federal government to address the sequelae of such tragic events by enacting the Disaster Relief Act of 1974. This was the first concerted and organized program designed to undertake what was needed for disaster relief. While a few ad hoc efforts were made to study emotional and mental problems occurring in disasters in the early 1970's, no systematic procedures were in place prior to 1976.

Legal Precedent

A precursor to PTSD as we presently know it was set forth in the courts in a trial over a three-year period. Although unable to provide sufficient discretionary money at the time it was needed, psychiatrists from the University of Cincinnati had contacted me at NIMH seeking funds to study the effects of a major disaster in West Virginia. That work then contributed, in part, to establishing the first legal precedent for the acceptance of psychic impairment resulting from disasters (Stern 1976). This occurred when the Pittston Mining company was held legally liable in the Buffalo Creek Dam disaster. The company's coal-waste refuse pile, which was used to dam a mountain stream, burst without warning in 1972, devastating sixteen small communities in the Buffalo Creek Valley where more than 125 people perished and 1,000 homes were destroyed. The settlement of $13.5 million provided $5.5 million for property loss and wrongful death damage payments with approximately $8 million set apart for psychic impairment. As a result, some 600 plaintiffs each recovered $13,000 for psychological injuries.

Loss of life in a community, however, is not correlated with the extent of psychological damage incurred. For example, when the Grand Teton Dam burst in 1976 and the Snake River overflowed in Southern Idaho, eleven persons lost their lives but crisis counseling services in six centers provided psychological counseling to more than 1000 subjects. A series of other disastrous events occurred during the 1970's in which this author became involved, along with my staff at NIMH.

Sociological and Psychological Issues

Early research in disasters during the 1950s focused upon such issues as engineering concerns, flood-plain management, mobility, housing problems and community organization. Work was carried out largely by engineers and sociologists, with the latter emphasizing the importance of disavowing what they believed to be erroneous prevailing beliefs. It was felt that prominent myths existed about irresponsible emotional reactions of victims which they believed should be dispelled. Instead, based upon a few short-term studies, they felt that in virtually every disastrous event, victims always behaved quite responsibly while putting their efforts into cohesive and constructive channels. A number of aphorisms were then set forth saying that looting did not occur in disaster but only in riots and people could be counted upon to become cohesive, cooperative and well focused. We now know that such is not the case, that looting is practically inevitable in major disasters, with the prevalence of wide spread anger and discontent. Moreover, a litany of psychophysiological reactions occur including sleep disturbances, anxiety and depression, along with marital disturbances, alcoholism and drug abuse (Frederick, 1977; Cohen & Ahearn, 1980).

Illustrative Salient Events

Among the catastrophic events occurring during this period were the following: the Sylmar earthquake in California in 1971, the Boston blizzard in 1977 where severe winter storms and flooding shut down a major metropolitan city for the first time, the Big Thompson Canyon flood in a resort area of Colorado in 1976, the Mt. St. Helens volcano in 1980 in Washington, and the Three Mile Island nuclear plant accident in Pennsylvania in 1979.

Although a number of the disasters occurred during my tenure at the NIMH, each with its own disheartenment and pathos, perhaps a particularly illustrative and dramatic event will be helpful in delineating the activities involved in such situations. The Three Mile Island (TMI) nuclear accident at Middletown, Pennsylvania, on March 28, 1979, occurred when equipment failure and human error led to a loss of coolant material and a partial meltdown in one nuclear reactor, resulting in the worst nuclear accident in US history. This momentous event precipitated the immediate involvement of a number of Federal and private agencies. Since this author was directing the NIMH program for Disaster Assistance and Emergency Health at the time, I was asked to serve as an on-site representative to provide information to the Secretary of Health Education and Welfare (now the Department of Health and Human Services).

The Governor of the Commonwealth of Pennsylvania, the Honorable Richard Thornburgh, established a Commission to provide a report on the various facets of the disaster, including health studies. An Advisory Panel to the Department of Health was formed. The Advisory Panel on Health Research Studies consisted of a distinguished group of scientists, chaired by Leroy Burney, M.D., former Surgeon General, and former President of the Milbank Memorial Fund. Thus, it became this author's honor to serve as the only member of the Federal government as well as the only psychologist appointed to that Panel. During that period he was also appointed to the National Institutes of Health - TMI Follow-up Research Subcommittee, chaired by Arthur Upton, M.D., Director of the National Cancer Institute, whose task it was to assess the biological effects of ionizing radiation. The radiation doses received by workers at the TMI plant from April 1 through April 15, 1979, while substantially greater than those received by the off-site population, were not demonstrably in excess of the maximum permissible annual dose limit of 5,000 mrem (Upton, 1979).

This author entered the plant on several occasions with minimal film badge readings. From film badges readings of 262 plant workers it appeared that all but seven received less than 1000 mrem, with the three largest doses recorded as 3000-4000 mrem. Hence, the detection of chromosome abnormalities attributable to the accident would be difficult, if not impossible, to prove. A cloud of radioactive material from the plant wafted its way over a field of cows, resulting in detectable doses of radioactivity in their milk for a few days following the accident. While it soon dissipated, there was concern since many foods contain milk, such as chocolate.

Several state-supported studies were carried out during that period. However, only three Federally approved studies were conducted: a) a study of pregnant women and their offspring by the Health Services Administration; b) a population registry survey by the Center for Disease Control; and c) a study by my office at NIMH through the epidemiology department at the University of Pittsburgh on the emotional and psychological effects upon 1200 persons in the TMI area and a companion plant in the western part of the State. At the end, the President's Commission and the Governor's Commission agreed that the only significant findings were psychological, noting "the major health effect of the accident appears to have been on the mental health of the people living in the region" (Governor's Report, p. 14, February 1980).

International collaborative projects could be stimulated through several avenues such as the Agency for International Development (AID) within the Department of State, Section 408 funds at the NIMH, and the Pan American Health Organization (PAHO). Section 408 funds are allocated for foreign travel for exploration of research collaboration with other countries. The author's own activities entailed work with authorities in Yugoslavia while at NIMH and in Central and South America as an Advisor to PAHO. Since that time there has been additional work into various aspects of violence and trauma with support from several private funding sources.

For a number of years, FEMA only supplied funding assistance for natural disasters. NIMH, however, came to realize the pressing and continuing needs for support into human-induced calamities.

At NIMH, research grant support can now come from three avenues under the Violence and Traumatic Stress Research Program, the Victims of Interpersonal Violence Research Program or the Violence and Traumatic Stress Research Branch. These units may supply funding for studies in such areas as family violence, rape, spousal abuse, as well as criminal violence, such as robbery, homicide, kidnapping and terrorism. In 1990, under Section 301 of Public Law 78-410, as amended, 42 US Code 241 (42 CFR part 52) subject to the availability of funds, support became accessible via the Rapid Assessment Post-Impact of Disaster plan (Burke & Judd, 1990). Grants became available to any public or nonprofit institution such as a university, college, hospital or community agency, unit of State or local government, and authorized units of the Federal Government, and to for-profit institutions and entities.

Today, the existence of deleterious emotional sequelae in varying degrees from a variety of disasters is greater than ever in all walks of life. During the 5.9 Whitier earthquake in 1987, the School of Dentistry building at UCLA had undergone tremendous shaking, which had elicited profound fear among professional staff. Knowledge of mental health disorders by professionals provided no immunity in time of personally perceived disaster. The earthquake in Southern California severely damaged my own home as well as those of other coworkers. Curiously, our personal conditioned responses to a 5.1 after-shock evoked broad-based instantaneous panic reactions. Such feelings are quite prevalent in light of such continuing after-shocks, thereby, requiring incident-specific and trauma-specific interventions, which the author has described in detail elsewhere (Frederick, 1987). Although FEMA supplied appreciable assistance for property damage and needed housing, psychological intervention was given largely by local resources. It should be noted that while much progress has been made in supporting psychological work, it is apt to be viewed as a lesser priority in the scheme of things to address. Its importance often gets short shrift, particularly during periods of personnel retrenchment, shrinking resources and fiscal austerity.

Self-knowledge and self-improvement are very difficult for most people.
It usually needs great courage and long struggle.

Abraham Maslow

Traumatic Stress Centers and Their Role in Knowledge
of
Post-Disaster States

Jacob Lindy, MD
Bonnie Green, PhD
Mary Grace, M.Ed., MS

Following World War II, Kiardiner (1947) lamented the status of psychiatric knowledge in the area of trauma responses after natural disaster, war and industrial accidents. He pointed out that research into the area of pathogenesis and service delivery was hampered by the absence of centers committed to continuous, programmatic research. In fact, what characterized previous work was that a group finding itself exposed to a disaster studied that event, but in isolation from others. At the time, we lacked a common diagnostic language, common instruments to measure pathology, or empirical models to assess longitudinal outcome. One of the major factors contributing to the acceleration of trauma work in the past two decades has been the presence of university-based trauma research ventures where that research has been continuous over time.

Among the earlier centers was one in Oslo, Norway, where the work of Eitinger, et al., with World War II prison camp survivors (1973) was followed by the work of Weiseaths, et al., with North Sea survivors, UN peacekeeping casualties. Another was in Cincinnati where interest in occupational trauma, WWII trauma, and Holocaust trauma set the state for intensive examination of survivors of the Buffalo Creek Dam collapse (Gleser et al., 1981; Titchener, 1976). The authors, in the second generation of investigators (Green, Grace and Lindy) gave the center a formal name and set out on a course of programmatic research.

Beginning in 1974, the University of Cincinnati Traumatic Stress Study Center became one of the early university-based clinical research teams to investigate the psychiatric impact of disaster in a programmatic way. Initially, the authors' interests were in predicting survivors at risk for more long-term pathology following trauma, in devising secondary prevention and treatment strategies and in measuring outcome results.

The authors' participation began on a stormy day in March of 1974, while they were headed to Buffalo Creek to evaluate some 200 survivors of the Buffalo Creek Dam collapse which had occurred in 1972. There in the heart of deep coal country of Appalachia, the authors first saw an epidemic of PTSD at a time before the diagnosis was established. Periodic returns to the valley have now given data over a 20-year span on these trauma survivors. Upon returning to Cincinnati in March 1974, the authors learned that tornadoes had hit just north and west of Cincinnati shortly after their departure for Buffalo Creek. Clinical descriptions and research studies of these two sites primed the authors to be more responsive so that in May, 1977, when a giant supper club burned down south of the city, killing 165, the authors were well-positioned to respond, and begin their activities the night of the fire at a temporary morgue. This effort continued through outreach, clinical treatment and a two-year follow-up study.

In 1979, the local outreach officer of the Disabled American Veterans (DAV) introduced the authors to the many returning Vietnam Veterans in the community whose pathology was so reminiscent of the other groups with which the authors worked. After setting up the first rap group for Vietnam Veterans in the area, there was a follow-up of 200 Vietnam Veterans for over one year, with fifty enrolled in a treatment project.

In addition to the widening spectrum of these major studies and treatment projects, the authors worked with survivors of a crush of 15 people outside a rock concert by the group "Who," with survivors of a Canadian Airlines plane crash victims, an explosion at a chemical plant in the city and recipients of the unexpected news of unintentional exposure to long-term low-grade exposure to radioactive contamination from a nuclear armaments plant near Cincinnati.

As the authors' efforts grew, they networked with other investigators and soon found themselves playing several roles in a developing field:

1. Describing the phenomenology of PTSD and establishing it as a valid diagnosis.
2. Designing a model for understanding contributing factors in long-term outcome of exposure to trauma.
3. Describing the long-term course of illness.
4. Delineating problems in outreach.
5. Developing models and techniques for on-site activity for mental health practitioners to differing traumatic events.
6. Facing challenges in mobilizing incident-specific responses.
7. Describing characteristic phases of treatment.
8. Reporting reactions of therapists engaged in such treatments.
9. Studying the outcome of intervention.

Once the authors determined the basic stressor unit, there was a considerable generalizability across disasters. Being aware of the many confounding variables to be considered in each disaster situation was valuable.

Out of the aforementioned work, the authors have come to see the mental health professionals as having several important roles. First, at the local level, members of the mental health response team need to become members of civic disaster planning efforts so that when disaster strikes they are known co-workers with medical teams, Red Cross, pathologists, crisis clergy and others likely to be on the trauma scene. Second, at the disaster site, specially prepared mental health workers can play important roles in limiting access to disfigured bodies. Third, mental health professionals can join the media in efforts to inform, educate and influence a positive recovery climate for the traumatized, including consultations to community leaders, assistance in designing memorials and establishing special anniversary events. Mental health workers can follow-up with survivors, rescue workers and families, and devise longer-term strategies for outreach to an interventions with survivors especially at risk.

Differing elements in the trauma configuration affected the form and onset of pathological reactions. Acute reactions were most affected by threat to life and traumatic loss. Delayed reactions developed more with exposure to the grotesque. Anxious and depressive features of the syndrome were associated with the former elements and addictive disorders with the second. Community disruption increased severity and delayed recovery.

Through longitudinal studies, the authors confirmed the field's notion (after 1980) that PTSD could indeed be a chronic disorder. Roughly 20 years after trauma, survivors at Buffalo Creek showed a PTSD rate of 30%, although the intensity of the disorder was much muted (Green, et al.).

Ways of coping with the trauma affected outcome, as in taking initiatives in clean-up activities at Buffalo Creek which promoted mastery unless such activity exposed survivors to further grotesque images such as buried body parts. Problem-solving, affect expression and activating a network of emotional support all help, unless the trauma is exposure to radioactive contaminants or Agent Orange where cognition problem-solving makes things worse.

The climate for recovery influences rate of healing. Victims blamed for carrying out a dirty war (Vietnam), or behaving like barbarians at a rock concert (the Who concert), or stigmatized in their exposure to radioactivity (Fernald) do less well than those whose family and community take in their wounds as their own. Psychotherapy, or even formal research or interviews themselves may be seen as one more salutary effect folded within the recovery environment, in that putting the experience to words seems to help.

Psychotherapists specially acculturated to the circumstances of the trauma are more effective than those unaware of such details. More seasoned practitioners are more effective. Supervision in a planned manner improves results. Modalities selected may be less important than the comfort practitioners have in using them.

The relationship with the therapist becomes an important fulcrum around which the work of resolving trauma rests. The survivor is reluctant to seek help and distrustful of those who intrude. But, once the survivor draws the therapist within his trauma membrane, the relationship becomes intense, although sometimes still brittle. Maintaining the working alliance requires consistent attention to the trauma in how it may be repeating itself and with special emphasis on the ethics of the relationship. The survivor learns to master damaged trust first by learning to trust the therapist.

The emotional experiences of the therapist as he or she engages the survivor and the trauma story is immense. It is at this point where treatments are most fragile and where the therapist can unwittingly push the survivor away, or over-identify, leaving significant pieces of the work of therapy unaddressed.

Finally, the authors have attempted to include outcome studies with their work. Thus, the authors may say that survivors who are able to engage in a dynamic psychotherapeutic process and complete a planned termination will improve significantly, both in the intrusive and the numbering components of the illness. Such improvement is measurable within the first 18 months after a disaster and even when the treatment occurs as long as 15 years afterward. Further, some of the improvement in numbering and alienation is not achieved by psychopharmacology alone.

Today, the authors, from the original University of Cincinnati Traumatic Stress Study Center, look across their shoulders at the numerous high quality university-based clinical and research centers at Duke, UCLA, Yale, Stanford, Harvard, Dartmouth, South Carolina, Langley-Porter and Cleveland State. These centers focus their work on individual cases of PTSD, but by being on the spot when large-scale natural and community disaster strikes, are able to contribute in a systematic way to the knowledge of survivors of natural disaster and the ability to react forcibly and positively to their plight.

Nature's worst brings out humanity's best.

Bill Clinton, President
1995

World Federation for Mental Health (WFMH)

Kathleen Allden, MD

The World Federation for Mental Health (WFMH), founded in 1948, is the only international non-governmental coalition of professionals, volunteers and consumers accredited as a consultant in mental health to all of the United Nations' major agencies. Its goal is the promotion of the mental health of "all of the world's peoples." Those whose mental health is at greater risk are people forced to leave their homes and find shelter and security elsewhere - among strange people, strange places, strange languages and customs. WFMH, which has individual and organizational members in over 110 countries and offices at the UN in New York, Geneva and Paris, plays a vital role in addressing mass disasters in the vastly expanding refugee problem in the changing geopolitical context of the post-Cold War era.

At the beginning of 1993, the United Nations High Commissioner for Refugees (UNHCR) estimated that there were 18.2 million refugees worldwide; and that to reach that number an average of 10,000 people per day were forced to leave their countries during the previous year for fear of persecution, violence and other natural disasters. According to a UNHCR document (1993), UNHCR estimates there are an additional 24 million people displaced within their own borders. These numbers are astonishing in view of the fact that there were only 4.6 million refugees as recently as 1978. The numbers continue to swell: tragedies such as the one in Rwanda have broken out in every major geopolitical region. Most refugees, especially the internally displaced, live in abject poverty; only a fraction receive protection and assistance from the international community. Mrs. Sadaka Ogata, UNHCR, recently stated:

"As the world gropes for a new political and economic equilibrium, as historic hatreds are unleashed, as old power structures crumble and new ones are yet to be formed, as the gap between the rich and the poor widens, as demographic pressure grows, the phenomenon of displacement has taken on frightening proportions, as much within the borders as across them (Ogata, 1993)."

227

Complicating the loss of home and fear of persecution is the fact that many refugees have experienced torture. Various studies estimate that 5 to 35% of refugees have been tortured (Baker, 1992). At the same time, the refugee field is moving beyond the initial strict definition of human rights abuse and proposing a broadening of the interpretation to include social and cultural rights and the physical and psychosocial consequences of these violations. The implication of this evolution is the necessity of providing rehabilitation to refugees at the individual, family, community and societal levels. But, before this can be done, the trauma must be understood within the unique cultural and political context of the particular society and individual. For example, sexual violence and rape will have varying social consequences for a woman depending on her cultural group.

Refugee policies developed in the aftermath of World War II and expanding as a result of Cold War tensions require restructuring. Refugee policy is shifting away from resettlement in developed countries and confinement camps, as the Cambodians experienced for over a decade, to resolution and prevention of crises within the countries of origin, as in the former Yugoslavia. The violence of war, civil conflicts and genocidal policies continue to create additional highly traumatized populations (Rogers, 1992). The serious impact on the mental health and social functioning of traumatized refugees confined to camps for extended periods of time is being scientifically clarified (Molica et al., 1993). Now thinking is emerging which admits there is a wide gap between traditional refugee assistance based on food-water-shelter and the need for intelligent development programs which recognize the need for population-based interventions to address the sequelae of severe mass violence and displacement. A 1992 report on repatriation and development by an executive committee of UNHCR (1992) states:

"...it has become clear that there exists a serious gap between relief assistance and development programs. This gap not only threatens the successful reintegration of returnees in terms of their ability to remain home and to rebuild their lives, it also threatens the viability of their communities."

World Federation for Mental Health
and the
First International Committee on Refugees and Migrants

In 1986, WFMH established with its collaborating center, the Harvard Program in Refugee Trauma (HPRT), a division of the Harvard School of Public Health, established the first International Committee on Refugees and Migrants. Membership on that committee includes individuals (many of them refugees) from all major regions of the world affected by refugee crises. Because of the groundbreaking work of the WFMH/HPRT collaboration, in June 1993, the High Commissioner of UNHCR signed an historic memorandum of agreement with WFMH/HPRT expanding the traditional advisory role of WFMH and adding a focal point for mental health within UNHCR. WFMH/HPRT is positioned to provide professional evaluation of psychosocial/mental health programs being considered by UNHCR and on-site consultation regarding refugee psychosocial/mental health emergencies.

The pioneering WFMH/HPRT collaboration is grounded in four essential areas: clinical care of the traumatized mentally-disturbed refugee, research, training and public policy. HPRT's clinical affiliate, the Indochinese Psychiatry Clinic (OPC), was established in Boston, Massachusetts in 1981 to meet the mental health needs of newly resettled, highly traumatized Cambodian, Vietnamese, Lao and Hmong refugees. IPC developed the Bicultural Model of psychiatric treatment which joins western clinicians with Indochinese mental health specialists in a multidisciplinary and culturally sensitive approach to mental health care. IPC has served as a model for newly established clinics in Australia, New Zealand, Italy, India (Tibetan) and Southeast Asia. The clinic also serves as a training site for physicians, psychology and social work students and graduate students of public health.

WFMH/HPRT served as consultant to the UN Border Relief Operation (UNBRO) to ameliorate the suffering and mental health problems of the more than 400,00 Cambodians who were confined to camps at the Thai-Cambodian border from 1986 until repatriation in 1993. In 1990, UNBRO granted WFMH/HPRT permission to conduct a landmark study of the health, mental health and social function of the residents of 1000 households in the Site 2 refugee camp at the Thai-Cambodian border. The findings of this study together with other HPRT studies of refugee communities in Asia and the U.S. indicate that traumatized refugee populations are extremely resilient; only a small percentage are susceptible to developing serious mental illness. The studies also indicate the necessity of identifying high-risk groups such as victims of sexual violence and torture, the physically handicapped, widows, abused children, the mentally ill, and the mentally retarded in order to formulate meaningful refugee programs. Acknowledging the limitations of cross-sectional analyses and in order to understand the phenomenon of the refugee's experience, HPRT's scientific work draws on the expertise of many fields such as psychiatry and psychology, anthropology, history, the other social sciences and epidemiology.

During 1992, in anticipation, WFMH/HPRT conducted a mental health training program in Site 2 for 60 Cambodian refugees to help prepare them to address the mental health needs of their home communities in Cambodia. The trainees were certified as Family-Child Mental Health Workers (FCMHW) by WFMH/HPRT. In April 1994, HPRT, under the auspices of the Ministry of Health of Cambodia, established a mental health training program in Cambodia known as the Harvard Training Program in Cambodia (HTPC). FCMHWs trained at the border by HPRT and other qualified Cambodian nationals have been recruited to work with primary care physicians to provide mental health services. Primary care physicians and FCMHWs receive supervision and consultation from the Boston-based team as well as the HTPC center located in Siem Reap Province.

In June 1993, in Utrecht, the Netherlands, HPRT collaborated with UNHCR and a group of twenty-five Eastern and Western European mental health professionals to develop and establish the basic principles for providing for the care and rehabilitation of victims of rape, torture and other traumas in former Yugoslavia. In the fall of 1994, HPRT launched a mental health screening and training program in former Yugoslavia. In 1995 HPRT launched a program of new mental health initiatives in former Yugoslavia which focus on training in the evaluation and treatment of related disorders for health and mental health professionals, primary care physicians and educators.

In the coming century the world will face increasingly complex disasters resulting in additional massive upheavals of large populations. Expertise from diverse scientific disciplines will be required to develop policies and programs which move beyond the concept of providing food-water-shelter and (1) resolve conflicts and prevent large scale displacement; (2) emphasize human development of traumatized populations and the return to autonomy and economic self-sufficiency for the large numbers facing repatriation; (3) avoid prison-like conditions in refugee camps, minimize the time spent in camps and dependency on care providers for those who are forced to live in refugee camps. WFMH has members from widely diverse disciplines with a wealth of professional knowledge and expertise who share a common interest in promoting the mental health of those who are at greatest risk. WFMH remains uniquely qualified to serve as an advisory and consultative body to governmental and international organizations charged with the responsibility of caring for displaced persons within or outside of their national boundaries.

APPENDICES

APPENDIX A

Selected List of Agencies For Disaster Assistance

Adventist Community Services
Andrews University
Berrien Springs, MI 49104
Phone: (800) 253-3000

Brother to Brother International
824 Grandview Avenue
Pitsburgh, PA 15211
Phone: (412) 481-4798

American Jewish Joint Distribtion Committee
JDC International Development Program
711 Third Avenue
New York, NY 10017
Phone: (212) 687-6200
Fax: (212) 370-5467
Telex: 62873

CARITAS International, Inc.
PO Box 10-0179
Brooklyn, NY 11210
Phone: No Phone

American Red Cross Disaster Relief
PO Box 9140
Church Street Station
New York, NY 10256
Phone: (212) 875-2068
Fax: (212) 875-2357

Catholic Relief Services
PO Box 17090
Baltimore, MD 21298-9644
Phone: (800) SEND-HOPE
Fax: (410) 625-2220

AMERICARES Foundation
51 Locust Avenue
New Cannan, CT 06840
Phone: (800) 486-HELP
Fax: (203) 966-5195

Catholic Charities USA
Disaster Response
1731 King Street, Suite 200
Alexandria, VA 22314
Phone: (703) 549-1390

Black American Response to the African Crisis
261 E. Colorado Boulevard, Suite 210
Pasadena, CA 91101
Phone: (800) 584-0303

Change for God
2439 Ontario Road NW
Washington, D.C. 20009
Phone (202) 328-6922

Box Project
PO Box 435
Plainville, CT 06062
Phone: (203) 747-8182

Christian Children's Fund
203 E. Cary Street
Richmond, VA 23219
Phone: (800) 441-1000

Church World Service Aids for the Horn of Africa - c/o Church World Service
Natl. Council of Churches of Christ - USA
Africa Office, Room 612 475 Riverside Dr.
New York NY 10115
Phone: (212) 870-2645

Concern America
PO Box 1790
2024 N. Broadway, Sutie 205
Santa Ana, CA 92792
Phone: (714) 953-0857

Cooperative for Assistance and Relief Everywhere (CARE)
151 Ellis Street, NE
Atlanta, GA 30303-2439
Phone: (404) 681-2552
Fax: (404) 577-6075
For Info: (800) 422-7385
For Donations: (800) 521-CARE

CROP
PO Box 968
Elkhart, IN 46515
Phone: (219) 264-3102

Direct Relief Internations
27 South Lapatera Lane
Santa Barbara, CA 93117
Phone: (805) 964-4767
Fax: (805) 681-4838
Emergency: (805) 963-2555

Disaster Relief Fund of B'nai B'rith
1640 Rhode Island Avenue, NW
Wahsington, DC 20036
Phone: (202) 857-6582

Federal Emergency Management Agency
PO Box 70274
Washington, DC 20472
Phone: (202) 646-4252 Fax:(202) 646-3923

Food for the Hungry
7729 E. Greenway Road
Scottsdale, AZ 85260
Phone: (800) 2-HUNGER

Inter-Lutheran Disaster Relief
8765 W. Higgins Raod
Chicago, IL 60631
Phone: (215) 395-6891

International Alert
Working for the Resolution of Conflict
1 Glyn Street
London SE11 5HT UK
Phone: 44-71-793-8383
Fax: +44 71-793-7975
E-Mail: INT-ALERT@geo2.geonet.de

Mennonite Central Committee
21 S 12th Street
PO Box 500
Akron, PA 17501-0500
Phone: (717) 859-1151

OXFAM AMERICA
26 West Street
Boston, MA 02111-1206
Phone: (617) 482-1211
Fax: (617) 728-2594

Presiding Bishop's Fund for World Relief, The
815 Second Avenue
New York, NY 10017
Phone: (212) 922-5129 or (800) 334-7626
FAX: (212) 983-6377

Salvation Army World Service Office
PO Box 269
615 Slaters lane
Alexandria, VA 22313
Phone: (703) 684-5500
Fax: (703) 684-3478

Save the Children
PO Box 975
Westport, CT 06881
Phone: (203) 221-4000

United Methodist Committee on Relief
PO Box 5050
Church Street Station
New York, NY 10249
Phone: (212) 870-3600

US Committee for UNICEF, The
333 E. 38th Street
New York, NY 10016
Phone: (212) 686-5522

World Concern
PO Box 33000
Seatle, WA 98133
Phone: (906) 546-7201

World Vision
PO Box 1131
Pasadena, CA 91131
Phone: (800) 777-5777

APPENDIX B

Selected List of Professional Associations and Institutes

American Orthopsychiatric Association
330 Seventh Avenue
18th Floor
New York, NY 10001
Phone: (212) 564-5930
FAX: (212) 564-6900

Earthquake Engineering Research Institute
499 14th Street
Suite 320
Oakland, CA 94612-1902
Phone: (415) 451-0905
Fax:　(415) 451-5411

Arts and Community University of South Florida
Tampa, FL 33620
Phone: (813) 974-3168

European Centre for Disaster Medicine
La Pantiere
1261 Bogis-Bossey
Switzerland
Phone:
Fax:　+4122-776-64-17

International Association of Trauma Counselors, Inc. (IATC)
1033 La Posada Drive
Suite 220
Austin, TX 78752-3880
Phone: (512) 454-8626
Fax:　(512) 454-3036

International Society for Traumatic Stress Studies (ISTSS)
60 Revere Dr., Suite 500
Northbrook, IL 60062
Phone: (708) 480-9028
Fax:　(410) 480-9282

Listen to the Children - Cooperative Disaster Child Care Program
500 Main Street
PO Box 188
New Windsor, MD 21776-0188
Phone: (410) 635-8734
Fax:　(410) 635-8739

Meteorological & Geoastrophysical Abstracts
c/oMGA Inforonics, Inc.
550 Newtown Road
PO Box 458
Littleton, MA 01460-0458
Phone: (508) 486-8976
Fax:　(508) 486-0027

National Organization For Victim Assistance (NOVA)
1757 Park Road, NW
Washington, DC 20010
Phone: (202) 232-6682
FAX: (202) 462-2255

National Center for PTSD Women's Health Sciences Division VA Medical Center (116B-3)
150 South Huntington Avenue
Boston, MA 02130
Phone: (617) 232-9500 Ext 5916, 4145
Fax:　(617) 278-4515

National Crisis Prevention Institute, Inc.
3315-K North 124th Street
Brookfield, WI 53005
Phone: (800) 558-8976 (414) 783-5787
Fax: (414) 783-5906

National Library of Medicine
Bethesda MD 20894
Phone: (301) 496-0508
Fax: (301) 480-3035
E-mail: TLC@1hc.nlm.nih.gov

Society for Applied Sociology (SAS)
c/o Management Support Services, Inc.
1117 East Spring Street
New Albany, IN 47150
Phone: (812) 944-1826

Traumatic Stress Institute
22 Morgan Frams Drive
South Windsor, CT 06074-1369
Phone: (203) 644-2541
Fax: (203) 644-6891
Email: CAAPTSI@AOL.com

**Trauma Recovery Education and
Counseling Center**
9 North Third Street
Suite 100 #14
Warrenton, VA 22186
Phone: (703) 341-7339
Fax: (703) 341-7339

**University of Delaware
Disaster Research Center**
77 E. Main St.
Newark, DE 19716
Phone: (302) 831-2000
FAX: (302) 831-2091

University of Wisconsin
Dept. of Governmental Affairs
Mitchell Hall, Room 215
PO Box 413
Milwakee, WI 53201
Phone: (414) 229-4753
Fax: (414) 229-6930

**The World Association for Disaster
and Emergency Medicine (WADEM)**
1947 Camino Vida Roble
Suite 203
Carsbad, CA 92008
Phone: (619) 431-6975
Fax: (619) 431-8135 or (619) 431-8176

The World Federation for Mental Health
1021 Prince Street
Alexandria, VA 22314-2971
Phone: (703) 838-7543
Fax: (703) 684-5968

APPENDIX C

Selected List of Disaster Publications and Journals

1. US Government Printing Office (1992). The Federal Response Plan (For Public Law 93-288, as amended). Washington, D.C.: FEMA 229

2. Frederick, C., and Farberous (1978). NIMH Training Manual for Human Service Workers in Major Disasters.

3. Art from Ashes, Bay Area Arts Relief Project. c/o Cultural Arts Division, 474 14th Street, Suite 1130, Oakland, CA 94612.

4. School Intervention Following a Critical Incident, Project COPE, FEMA 220/November 1991.

5. How to Help Children After a Disaster, FEMA 219/November 1991.

6. Crisis Intervention and Time-Limited Treatment. *Journal for Crisis Intervention*. Langhorne, PA: Harwood Academic Press. US (800) 545-8398; Fax: (215) 750-6343.

7. National Mental Health Association, Information Center. *Handling Disaster-Related Stress*. 1021 Prince Street, Alexandria, VA 22314-2971. (800) 969-6642.

8. Trauma Recovery Publications, workbooks, assessments and training seminars. PO Box 6689, Columbus, GA 31907.

9. *International Journal of Stress Management*. Human Science Press, Inc. 233 Spring Street, New York, NY 10013-1578, (800) 221-9369 Fax: (212) 807-1047.

APPENDIX D

DISASTER RELATED HANDOUTS

Critical Incident Symptoms
What To Look For
For Survivors and Their Families

A critical incident creates a stressor outside the realm of usual human experience. As a victim of this type of stress, you can expect to experience the after effects to varying degrees. We also want to alert you to the fact that there is a ripple effect through your family, loved ones and also your co-workers. The acknowledgment of these emotional reactions helps to shorten recovery time and prevent complications through the natural healing process.

Sense that life is out of balance

Disbelief

Flashbacks

Sleep Disturbance

Sadness

Diminished or Increased Sexual Drive

Minimization of the Critical Incident

Anger/Irritability

Forgetfulness

Cold-like Symptoms

Survivor Guilt

Increased Substance Use

Social Withdrawal

Emotional Numbing

Feelings of Being "Out of Control" or Fears of "Going Crazy

Loss of Feeling Secure in the World

Self-doubt

Greater Belief in Superstitions and Predictions

Hypervigilence, ie. constantly watching or listening for danger signs

Prepared by California Psychological Association

Critical Incident Symptoms
What To Do

If you are experiencing any of the above symptoms, the following techniques may be of help. Do not hesitate to make contact with professional mental health services if these symptoms persists or get worse.

Good nutrition which includes less processed foods, less salt, less sugar, less caffeine and more fruits and vegetables.

Adequate sleep and exercise.

Avoid major projects (including starting a new diet or quitting smoking).

Keep a familiar routine with familiar people and surroundings.

Don't push thoughts and memories of the event away. Go ahead and talk and talk or write or draw or compose or use some other form of self expression in order deal with your feelings.

Watch only enough TV to get information; don't traumatize yourself with it.

Use humor, tell jokes, watch comic videos, etc., (be sensitive).

Do some volunteer work.

Use positive self-talk such as "I am doing fine, things will get better."

Encourage and support co-workers, make a conscious effort at compliments and teamwork.

When feeling tense or upset, take at least ten deep breaths and repeat as necessary.

Don't be embarrassed about a repetitious need to talk, be aware that some may not be able to listen to you because of their own emotional state.

Help yourself and others by joining a support group.

Take time out for fun, do something you have been wanting to do.

Take a hot bubble bath, read a good book, or listen to good music.

Take a break. Allow yourself time for pleasant fantasies, previous wonderful experiences or future exciting or interesting plans.

Participate in debriefings if available (A debriefing is an official assessment and evaluation of the situation and emotions).

If you feel you still need more help, seek professional assistance.

Prepared by California Psychological Association

HELPING YOUR CHILD AFTER A DISASTER

Children may be especially upset and show feelings about the disaster. These reactions are normal and usually will not last long. Listed below are some problems you may see in your children.

* Excessive fear of darkness, separation or being alone
* Clinging to parents; fear of strangers
* Worry
* Increase in immature behaviors
* Not wanting to go to school
* Changes in eating/sleeping behaviors
* Increase in aggressive behavior or shyness
* Bedwetting or thumbsucking
* Persistent nightmares
* Headaches or other physical complaints

Some things that will help your child are:

* Talk with your child about his/her feelings about the disaster. Share your feelings, too.
* Talk about what happened; give your child information he/she can understand.
* Reassure your child that you are safe and together. You may need to repeat this reassurance often.
* Hold and touch your child often.
* Spend extra time with your child at bedtime.
* Allow your child to mourn or grieve over a lost toy, a lost blanket, a lost home.
* If you feel your child is having problems at school, talk to his/her teacher so you can work together to help your child.

Please take this sheet with you today to re-read in the coming months. Usually a child's emotional response to a disaster will not last long. But some problems may be present or recur many months afterward. If you need further assistance, please call your local department of mental health.

Prepared by California Psychological Association

SAMPLE RADIO PUBLIC SERVICE ANNOUNCEMENTS
(POST-DISASTER)

Local media play a very important role in disaster. Before the disaster, they announce the possibility of its occurrence, give early warnings and instructions on evacuation, and provide information on injury prevention and loss or destruction of property. After the disaster, they may serve as invaluable information centers for locating victims, rumor control, availability of community resources and as a tangible source of hope for reconstruction and restoration of the community. The media are familiar agents in a community. The emotional impact of a large-scale disaster is one of chaos. Calm, clear instructions by the media help restore a sense of order and allow individuals and the community to regroup their energies with hope for the future.

The radio public service announcements included here will inform the public about emotional and daily living problems following a disaster. While some of the problems may be emotional in nature, they are not indicative of mental illness. Since embarrassment and taboo are still associated with mental illness, use of any terminology implying mental health problems should be avoided in the radio spots.

In addition, an interview might be arranged with an articulate representative of the mental health community on the anticipated emotional responses of disaster victims.

The most important points to make in a media campaign are:

* People in the community have undergone a traumatic, disruptive experience. It is normal to react with feelings of fear, anxiety, sorrow, anger, irritation, confusion and apathy. Physical ailments, sleep problems, appetite disturbances and apathy may result. Knowing these reactions are normal gives a person permission to bring such feelings into the open and deal with them. If these feelings persists, help should be sought.

* Since it's helpful to share these experiences and feelings, suggest that family, relatives, friends and neighbors talk with each other. Identify community resources where trained help is immediately available.

30-SECOND PUBLIC SERVICE ANNOUNCEMENT:

GENERAL

A disaster or catastrophe such as the (tornado, flood, fire) which struck our (area/town/community/city/region) recently, means **LOSS**: perhaps loss of relatives or friends, or loss of home and important belongings. Sometimes it means starting all over again. The emotional effects of these losses may show up immediately after a disaster or they may appear many months later. You may feel irritable or confused or you may suffer from headaches or insomnia. All these reactions are normal and usually pass quickly. But if these problems persist, call (phone number) for help in dealing with the disaster. Call (phone number).

CHILDREN

If you were frightened by the recent (tornado, flood, fire), think of your children. For them a disaster is a fearful force which has shaken their world out of control. Some children may regress to behaviors they had already outgrown, such as night terrors, a loss of toilet control, or clinging to parents. School-age children may refuse to attend school, withdraw, become irritable or exhibit unusual fears. If you are a parent, help your child rebuild a sense of security. This may mean spending extra time with your child, as you reassure and talk about your child's fears. If problems persist, help is available. Call (phone number). That's (repeat number).

Prepared by California Psychological Association

APPENDIX E

NATIONAL MENTAL HEALTH ASSOCIATION

Tips for Coping with Disaster

HANDLING DISASTER-RELATED STRESS

"I'm scared."
"I've felt strung out ever since the disaster."
"I can't seem to get my mind off this."
"I haven't slept at all since the disaster."
"How can I channel my frustration and anger into something constructive?"
"The destruction is all over television and paper and magazines - it leaves me depressed."

HOW DO I KNOW IF I'M EXPERIENCING NEGATIVE STRESS

Stress affects everyone differently. What mkay indicate negative stress inone person might just be a personality trait in another. In most cases, though, there are warning signs that indicate a need for active stress management.

These include:

> persistent fatigue
> inability to concentrate
> flashes of anger - lashing out at friends and family
> changes in eating and sleeping habits
> increased use of alcohol, tobacco, etc.
> prolonged tension headaches, lower backaches, stomach or other physical ailments
> prolonged feelings of depression, anxiety or helplessness

244

Things to Remember:

Stress is a normal reaction to disaster.

Negative stress can damage physical and mental health if not recognized and managed.

Things to Do:

Talk it out.

Try physical exercise.

Know your limits.

Take control.

Avoid self-medication.

Find a support group.

For more information, call:

National Mental Health Association
1-800-969-6642

Helping Children Handle Disaster-Related Anxiety

"I don't want to sleep alone."

"Mom and Dan are upset all of the time."

"I don't want to go to school."

PRE-SCHOOL AGE CHILDREN

Reassure pre-schoolers that they're safe.

Get a better understanding of a child's feelings about the disaster.

GRADE-SCHOOL AGE CHILDREN

False reassurance does not help this age group

Monitor children's media viewing

Allow them to express themselves through play or drawing

Don't be afraid to say "I don't know."

ADOLESCENTS

Encourage these youth to work out their concerns about the disaster. Adolescents may try to down-play their worries. It is generally a good idea to talk about these issues, keeping the lines of communication open and remaining honest about the financial, physical and emotional impact of the disaster on your family.

Things to Remember:

Be honest and open about the disaster.

Encourage children to express their feelings through talking, drawing or playing.

Children need comforting and frequent reassurance that they're safe make sure they get it.

UNDERSTANDING POST-TRAUMATIC STRESS DISORDER

It's been called shell shock, battle fatigue and war neurosis, but the disorder is not limited to soldiers. In the past, it was often misunderstood or misdiagnosed, but the disorder has very specific symptoms that together form a definite psychological syndrome.

POST-TRAUMATIC STRESS DISORDER
(PTSD)

- affects hundreds of thousands of people who have survived the trauma of natural disasters such as floods, accidental disasters, or deliberate, man-made disaster such as war;

- is an anxiety disorder that results from a terrifying, life-threatening event;

- can significantly interfere with a victim's ability to concentrate, to maintain close relationships with family and friends, and to function efficiently at a job;

- can contribute to the development of serious depressive illness and/or alcohol and substance abuse;

- can affect previously healthy, well-adjusted men, women, and children.

WHAT ARE THE SYMPTOMS OF PSTD?

- Vivid and sudden memories (flashbacks)
- Nightmares centering around the traumatic event.
- Avoidance phenomena
- Avoidance of accepting responsibility
- Exaggerated startle reactions
- Panic attacks

IS THERE TREATMENT FOR PSTD?

YES

- Individual Psychotherapy

- Family Therapy

- Peer Support Groups and "Rap" Groups

- Medications

Organizing a Mutual Support Group

"Where do I go to find others who know what I'm going through?"

"There must be some way for people like me to share experiences."

"I an't go through this alone."

Things to Do:

- Find out if a group for you already exists.
- Find a suitable location for your group meeting.
- Set the time.
- Plan outreach activities.
- Set the stage-plan the agenda, make seating arrangements, provide name tags, decide on refreshments and secure handouts.

For more information, call:

National Mental Health Association
1-800-969-6642

American Self-Help Clearing house
201-625-7101
TDD: 201-625-9053

National Self-Help Clearinghouse
212-642-2944

APPENDIX F

THE FEDERAL RESPONSE PLAN
Federal Emergency Management Agency
PO Box 70274
Washington, D.C. 20024

Federal resources are grouped into 12 **Emergency Support Functions** (ESF). Each is headed by a **Primary Agency.**

ESF 1: TRANSPORTATION
> **Responsibility:** Provide civilian and military transportation support.
> **Primary Agency:** Department of Transportation

ESF 2: COMMUNICATIONS
> **Responsibility:** Provide telecommunications support.
> **Primary Agency:** National Communications System

ESF 3: PUBLIC WORKS AND ENGINEERING
> **Responsibility:** Restore essential public services and facilities.
> **Primary Agency:** U.S. Army Corps of Engineers, Department of Defense

ESF 4: FIRE FIGHTING
> **Responsibility:** Detect and suppress wildland, rural and urban fires.
> **Primary Agency:** U.S. Forest Service, Department of Agriculture

ESF 5: INFORMATION AND PLANNING
> **Responsibility:** Collect, analyze and disseminate critical information to facilitate the overall Federal response and recovery operations.
> **Primary Agency:** Federal Emergency Management Agency

ESF 6: MASS CARE
> **Responsibility:** Manage and coordinate food, shelter and first aid for victims; provide bulk distribution of relief supplies; operate a system to assist family reunification.
> **Primary Agency:** American Red Cross

ESF 7: RESOURCE SUPPORT
> **Responsibility:** Provide equipment, materials, supplies and personnel to Federal entities during response operations.
> **Primary Agency:** General Services Administration

251

ESF 8: HEALTH AND MEDICAL SERVICES

Responsibility: Provide assistance for public health and medical care needs.

Primary Agency: U.S. Public Health Service, Department of Health and Human Services

ESF 9: URBAN SEARCH AND RESCUE

Responsibility: Locate, extricate and provide initial medical treatment to victims trapped in collapsed structures.

Primary Agency: Department of Defense

ESF 10: HAZARDOUS MATERIALS

Responsibility: Support Federal response to actual or potential releases of oil and hazardous materials.

Primary Agency: Environmental Protection Agency

ESF 11: FOOD

Responsibility: Identify food needs; ensure that food gets to areas affected by diseater.

Primary Agency: Food and Nutrition Service, Department of Agriculture

ESF 12: ENERGY

Responsibility: Restore power systems and fuel

Primary Agency: Department of Energy

APPENDIX G

International Decade for Natural Disaster Reduction

NATURAL DISASTER PREPAREDNESS

Preparedness means operation of a detection and warning infrastructure; dissemination of warnings and instructions; communication of information to and from communities before, during and after the disaster.

Prevention includes such mechanisms as development of scenarios of potential disasters; hazard mapping combined with assessing populations at risk; formulation of government policies and regulations; installation of detection and warning systems; land-use restrictions, environmental management such as reforestation and revegetation and application of structural engineering measures.

Are you prepared?

How about:
awareness of natural hazards around you?
emergency food supplies, medicines and water?
means of communications, e.g. radio?
house or building maintenance?
evacuation practices?

Is the community prepared?

How about:
emergency shelters?
emergency supplies?
means of alerting the community?
evacuationh plans?
training personnel to respond promptly?

Is the _Government_ prepared?

How about:
disaster prevention and mitigation programmes?
a national committee to assist preparedness-related programs and activites?
national co-ordination mechanisms?
public education campaigns?
relief and recovery activities?

Are the _business sector, scientific community and media_ involved?

How about:
financial and technical support for disaster management?
investment in infrastructure?
scientific and technological contributions?
early warning systems?
communications networks and co-ordination?

APPENDIX H

CALL FOR APPLICATIONS

ARMENIAN AMERICAN SOCIETY FOR STUDIES ON STRESS & GENOCIDE
IS SEEKING
EXPERTS IN MENTAL HEALTH FOR DISASTER OUTREACFH PROGRAM

Interested candidates please fill out the questionnaire below, and mail or fax as indicated:

NAME: (LAST NAME)_____(FIRST NAME)_____
ADDRESS:_____
        (CITY)_____(STATE)_____(ZIP)_____
TELEPHONE: (   )_____(please include area code)
FAX/E-MAIL: (   )_____(please include area code)

AFFILIATION:_____
ADDRESS:_____
        (CITY)_____(STATE)_____(ZIP)_____
TELEPHONE: (   )_____(please include area code)
FAX/E-MAIL: (   )_____(please include area code)

Highest Degree: Degree_____Date:_____Granting Institution:_____
Area of Specialization: Clinical: _____# of Years_____
                         Educational: _____# of Years_____
                         Research: _____# of Years_____
        Child:_____Adolescent:_____Adult:_____Older Adult:_____
COMPLETED RESEARCH:_____
ONGOING RESEARCH:_____
GRANTS RECEIVED:_____
PREVIOUS OUTREACH EXPERIENCE: Date:_____Place:_____
        Length of Time:_____
        Type of Involvement:_____
DISASTER TRAINING: INSTITUTION:_____
        Certification:_____
LANGUAGES:_____
AVAILABILITY:(Please specify the month, length of stay and notification requirements)

Please include your Curriculum Vitae and Supporting Articlies and return to:
Dr. Anie Sanentz Kalayjian, Co-Founder MHOP
130 West 79th Street, Suite 5E
New York, NY 10024
Phone: (212) 362-4018 or (201) 941-2266 Fax: (201) 941-5110

APPENDIX I

Selected Instrumentation in Stress, Trauma and Adaptation

Compassion Fatigue Self-Test for Practitioners

TYPE OF POPULATION: Adult. Human service field, generalizable to nearly any group including psychotherapists, teachers, public safety personnel, etc.

COST: Free

WHAT IT MEASURES: Addresses both trauma and burnout symptoms.

INSTRUMENT CONTENT SUMMARY: Burnout items taken from Pines (1993), trauma items gleaned from the trauma literature.

THEORETICAL ORIENTATION SUMMARY: integrative, but has roots in the Secondary Traumatic Stress literature.

Sample Items:

	Rarely Never	At Times	Not Sure	Often	Very Often
	1	2	3	4	5

I have thought I need more closr friends...
I have thought that htere is no one to talk with about
hightly stressful experience...
I have concluded that I work too hard for my own good...

INSTRUMENT CONTACT NAME: C.R. Figley, Ph.D.

Address:	Psychosocial Stress Research Program
	103 Sandels Hall, R86E
	Florida State University
	Tallahassee, Fl 32306
Phone:	904-644-1588
Fax:	904-644-4804
Email:	CFIGLEY@GARNET.ACNS.FSU.EDU

The Cultural Messages Scale

TYPE OF POPULATION: Women

COST: There is no cost to using the scale. We would greatly appreciate it if people who chose to use the scale would provide us with either summary data or the raw data that emerges from the use of the scale as this will facilitate further scale development.

INSTRUMENT CONTENT SUMMARY: the two versions of the scale (created to facilitate pre and post-testing) assess familiarity with, and endorsement of, common cultural constructions, (i.e. common beliefs, messages and ideas) about women, women and men, and sexuality. The scale includes items such as: "If you're not a virgin you're a whore; Women exist for men's sexual pleasure; A raped woman is soiled, damaged goods; A woman's attractiveness is her most important trait," etc. These, and other items were empirically derived from varied sources (focus groups of undergraduate students, media productions, transcripts of women who have been raped) and are intended to represent a fairly broad domain of cultural messages about women and sexuality. The scale is organized to evaluate both the subjects degree of familiarity with the items as well their agreement with the items on a five point interval rating format. Thus, for each item subjects familiar with, or recognize the item and, separately, the degree to which they agree or disagree with the content of the item. In addition to the actual scale items, the scale also contains a number of reversed sterotypes and positive statements intended to break response set and provide a way to evaluate the validity of an individual subjects score.

Sample Items:

Familiarity

1. not familiar to me
2. a little familiar to me
3. moderately familiar to me
4. fairly familiar to me
5. extremely familiar to me

Agreement

1. I strongly disagree
2. I somewhat disagree
3. I neither agree nor disagree
4. I somewhat agree
5. I strongly agree

Familiarity		Agreement

_____1.   A raped woman is soiled, damaged goods.   _____

_____2. Women should defer to male judgement in many matters. _____

_____3. Women can't act on their own sexual feelings because it _____
               is shameful or animalistic or selfish.

INSTRUMENT CONTACT NAME: Leslie Lebowitz, Ph.D.

Address: National Center for PTSD
Women's Health Sciences Division
(116B-2)
VAMC 150 S. Huntington Avenue
Boston, MA 02130

Phone: 617-232-9500 x4141 or leave message at
4145

Fax: 617-278-4501

Email: Lebowitz.Leslie@Boston.VA.Gov

Life Orientation Inventory (LOI)
Revision B

TYPE OF POPULATION: Adult/Adolescent

COST: Minimal

WHAT IT MEASURES: Aspects of spirituality along 5 dimensions.

INSTRUMENT CONTENT SUMMARY: Research version consists of 99 items (statements of belief)-Likert Rating Scale. Assess 5 dimensions of spirituality-attitude toward the non-material, awareness, hope, ontological relatedness, and meaning.

Sample Items:

1	2	3	4	5	6
Not at all true	Somewhat true	Moderately true	Quite true	Very true	Extremely true

_____1. I have had experiences which go beyond physical reality and rational thought.

_____2. There is life after death.

_____3. My life has meaning.

REFERENCES: Norms not yet established.

INSTRUMENT CONTACT NAME: Laurie Anne Pearlman, Ph.D.

Address:

The Traumatic Stress Institute
22 Morgan Farms Drive
South Windsor, CT 06074-1369

Phone: 203-644-2541
Fax: 203-644-6891
Email: CAAPTSI@AOL.com

259

Life Stressor Checklist

TYPE OF POPULATION:

COST: Minimal

WHAT IT MEASURES: The Life Stressor Checklist is a self-report instrument measuring the occurrence and impact of varying traumatic events across the life span.

INSTRUMENT CONTENT SUMMARY: The LSC addresses potentially traumatic events relating to: accidents and natural disasters; personal experiences; physical violence and assault; and sexual violence and assault. The instrument queries whether or not the event occurred, how upsetting it was at the time, how much it has affected the individual's life in the last year, and, where appropriate, whether life threat was experienced. Degree of the event's impact is measured on a 5 point Likert scale with 1 indicating no impact and 5 connoting extreme effects.

Sample Items:

1. Have you ever been emotionally abused or neglected (for example, being frequently shamed, embarrassed, ignored, or repeatedly told that you were 'no good')? **YES / NO**

2. Has someone close to you died suddenly or unexpectedly (for example, and accident, sudden heart attack, murder or suicide)? **YES / NO**

3. Have you ever seen a robbery, mugging, or attack taking place? **YES / NO**

REFERENCES:

Norris, F.H. (1992). Epidemiology of trauma: Frequency and impact of different potentially traumatic events on different demographic groups. *Journal of Consulting and Clinical Psychology*, 60, 400-408.

INSTRUMENT CONTACT NAME: Jessica Wolfe, Ph.D.

Address: National Center for PTSD
Women's Health Sciences Division

(116B-2)

VAMC 150 S. Huntington Avenue
Boston, MA 02130

Phone: 617-232-9500 x5916 or x4145
Fax: 617-278-4515

Los Angeles Symptom Check List (LASC)
[formerly the Foy, Sipprelle, Rueger, and Carrol Checklist]

TYPE OF POPULATION: any [has been used with combat veterans, battered women, adult survivors of childhood abuse, adolescent inner city gang members]

COST: Minimal

WHAT IT MEASURES: Symptoms of Post-traumatic Stress Disorder, plus associated features and complications.

INSTRUMENT CONTENT SUMMARY: The LASC consists of 43 brief phrases describing symptoms of PTSD or problems associated with it (e.g., difficulty concentrating, trouble trusting others, suicidal thoughts). The respondent is asked to supply a rating for each item, ranging from 0 (no problem) to 4 (extreme problem). There are three ways to score the instrument; (a) a sum of all 43 item ratings to obtain a global assessment of PTSD and accompanying indicators or general psychological distress; (b) a sum of the 17 items that most closely correspong to the dianostic criteria; and (c) a treichotomous classification as PTSD postive, partial PTSD, or PTSD negative as a function of the pattern of endorsements of these 17 items.

Sample Items:

0	1	2	3	4
No Problem	Slight Problem	Moderate Problem	Serious Problem	Extreme Problem

_____1. Trapped in an unsatisfying job.

_____2. Hostility/violence.

_____3. Dizziness/fainting

REFERENCES: There are a number of published studies by Foy and his associates, including:

Foy, Sipprelle, Rueger, and Carroll (1984). *Journal of Counsulting and Clinical Psychology*, 52.

Gallers, Foy, Donahoe, and Miller (1988). *Journal of Traumatic Stress*, 1.

Housekamp and Foy (1991). *Journal of Interpersonal Violence*, 6.

Resnick, Foy, Donahoe, and Miller (1989). *Journal of Traumatic Stress*, 45.

INSTRUMENT CONTACT NAME: David W. Foy, Ph.D.

Address: Graduate School of Education and
                                Psychology
                                Pepperdine University Plaza
                                400 Corporty Pointe
                                Culver City, CA 90230
Phone: 310-568-5739
Fax: 310-568-5755

NAME OF REVIEWER: Lynda and Dan King

Address: Department of Psychology,
                                Central Michigan University
                                Mt. Pleasant, MI 48859
Phone: 517-774-7589
Fax: 517-772-1497
Email: 3AJCQ3Q@CMUVM)

Psyhcobiological Assessment of PSTD

TYPE OF POPULATION: To date, primarily male veterans. Promising results exist for female sexual assault survives, sexually/physically abused children and vehicle accident survivors.

COST: Minimal

WHAT IT MEASURES:

Laboratory Abnormalities in PTSD

- Physiological assessment techniques
  - Psychophysiological Reactivity
  - Startle Response
  - EEG/Sleep Physiology
  - Event-Related Brain Potentials
- Baseline Neurohormone levels
  - catecholamines
  - cortisol
  - testosterone
  - thyroid
  - endophins
- Baseline receptor levels
  - lymphocyte glucocorticoid
  - Platelet alpha-2 adrenergic
  - Lymphocyte beta adrenergic
  - A_1-adenosine gustatory (panic>PTSD=normals)
- Challenge Tests
  - DST
  - yohimbine
  - MCPP
  - Stress-induced analgesia
    (with/without naloxone)
  - clonidine ® (growth hormone)
  - 1-DOPA ® (growth hormone)
  - CRF ® (ACTH)
  - TRH ® (TSH)
  - Odor-induced EEG

Feasible Psychobiological Approaches to Differential Diagnosis

Test	Comments
Psychophysiological Reactivity	Good distinction between PTSD and other anxiety disorders as well as MDD Hard to fake (may overlap with PD for neutral stimuli)
DST	Good distinction between PTSD, MDD (and normals) ?Any data on PD or anxiety disorders
Startle Response	Little comparative data between PTSD and other diagnosis Very robust response in PTSD
Unrinary Neurochormone Profiles	Clear distinction between PTSD and MDD Little data regarding PD or ansiety disorders
Yohimbine/Lactate	Should distinguish PTSD from MDD,not from PD
Thyroid Function tests	Elevated T_4 in PTSD More blunting of TRH in MDD?
Stress-induces analgesia	Should distinguish PTSD-needs to be tested (original finding needs to be replicated)
Sleep EEG	Laboratory findings too preliminary for clinical application
CRF	Laboratory findings too preliminary for clinical application
Growth Hormone Response (Clonidine, I-DOPA)	Laboratory findings too preliminary for clinical application
MCPP	Laboratory findings too preliminary for clinical application
Brain Imaging	Laboratory findings too preliminary for clinical application

INSTRUMENT CONTENT SUMMARY: Psychological Reactivity, Dexamethasome Suppression Test (DST), Startle response, Urinary Neurohormone Profiles, Thryoid Function Tests, Stress-induced analgesia.

REFERENCES:

Bremner, J.D. et al. (1993). Neurobiology of Post traumatic Stess Disorder. In: J.M. Oldham, M.B.. Riba and A. Tagman (eds.), *Review of Psychiatry*, volume 12. Washington, D.C., American Psychiatric Press, Inc.

Pitman, R.K. et al. (1987) Psychophysiologic assessment of post traumatic stress disorder imagery in Vietnam combat veterans. *Archives of General Psychiatry*, 44:970-9753.

Yehuda, R. et al. (1993) Enhanced suppression of cortisol following a low dose of dexamethasome in combat veterans with post traumatic stress disorder. *American Journal of Psychiatry* 150:83-96.

INSTRUMENT CONTACT NAME: Matthew J. Friedman M.D., Ph.D.

Address:	National Center for PTSD (116-D)
	VA Medical Center
	White River Junction, VT 05009
Phone:	802-296-5132
Fax:	802-296-5135
Email:	Mathw.Friedman@Dartmouth.Edu

Structured Interview for Measurement
of Disorders of Extreme Stress

TYPE OF POPULATION: Victims of interpersonal trauma, illness, disaster, and combat

COST: None

WHAT IT MEASURES: Alterations in regulation of affect, attention or consciousness, self-perception, relations with others, somatization, systems of meaning.

INSTRUMENT CONTENT SUMMARY: Using structured interview format, this measure evaluates 27 criteria often seen in response to extremely traumatic events. the instruments is designed to be used onloy in conjunctionwith a structured measure assessing the presence of PTSD/

AREAS EXAMINED:

I. Alterations in regulation of affect and impulses.
II. Alterations in attention or consciousness.
III. Alterations in Self-perception.
IV. Alterations in perception of the peroetrator.
V. Alterations in relations with others.
VI. Somatogation
VII. Alterations in systems of meaning

REFERENCES:

A structured interview for measurement of Disorders of Extreme Stress; submitted manuscript: Pelcovitz, van der Kolk, Roth, et. al.: contains summary of reliability information on this measure.

INSTRUMENT CONTACT NAME: David Pelcovitz, Ph.D.

Address: North Shore Hospital
Department of Psychiatry
300 Community Drive
Manhassett, NY 11030

Phone: 516-562-3005

Fax: 516-562-3997

INSTRUMENT CONTACT NAME: Bessel van der Kolk, M.D., Ph.D.

Address: Trauma Clinic
Mass. General Hospital
Harvard Medical School
25 Staniford Street
Boston, MA 02114

Phone: 617-727-5500-949

Fax: 617-248-0630

Trauma Ethics Questionnaire

TYPE OF POPULATION: Adult. Professional and Client

COST: Free

WHAT IT MEASURES: The TEQ addresses attitudes, values, beliefs, practices, and concerns in the area of ethical provision of treatment, research, training, and education. The instrument is also being used as tool for assessing what should be included in an ethical code for working with trauma survivors.

Sample Items:

5	4	3	2	1	0	NA
Always	Almost Always	Sometimes	Occas.	Rarely	Never	Don't Know NA

_____1. The locus of responsibility for effective treatment lies with the therapist.

_____2. Therapists are susceptible to secondary Post-traumatic stress reactions.

_____3. Working with PTSD leads to vicarious traumatization of therapists.

REFERENCES:

Williams, M.B., Sommer, J.F., Stamm, B.H.,. (in press). the development of ethical principles for post traumatic research, practice, training and publication. In M.B. Williams & J.F. Sommer, (eds). *Handbook of Post Traumatic Therapy.*

Williams, M.B., Sommer, J.F., Stamm, B.H.,.(1993). Developing ethical principles for Trauma Research, Education and Treatment.. Presented at the Ninth Annual Meeting of The International Society for Traumatic Stress Studies, Los Angeles, CA.

Williams, M.B., Sommer, J.F., Stamm, B.H., Harris, C.J. & Hammarberg, M. (1992). Developing ethical priniciples for the ISTSS-II: Developing comprehensive guidelines. Symposium presented at the Eighth Annual Meeting of The International Society for Traumatic Stress Studies, Los Angeles, CA.

Williams, M.B., Sommer, J.F., Stamm, B.H.,.(1992). Establishment of a Code of Ethics for the International Society for Traumatic Stress Studies.

Symposium presented at the First World Conference of The International Society for Traumatic Stress Studies, Amsterdam, The Netherlands.

Williams, M.B., Sommer, J.F., Stamm, B.H.,.(1991). Developing ethical principles for the ISTSS: Developing comprehensive guidelines. Symposium presented at the Eighth Annual Meeting of The International Society for Traumatic Stress Studies. Washington, D.C.

Williams, M.B., Sommer, J.F.,.(1990). Ethics and Trauma: Presented in The Research and Methodology Interest Group Pre-Meeting Institute of Sixth Annual Meeting of The International Society for Traumatic Stress Studies. Washington, D.C.

INSTRUMENT CONTACT NAME: Mary Beth Williams, Ph.D.

Address:	Trauma Recovery Education and Counseling Center
	9N. 3rd
	Suite 100 #14
	Warrenton, VA 22186
Phone:	703-341-7339
Fax:	703-241-7613

TSI Belief Scale, Revision L

TYPE OF POPULATION: Adults

COST: None

WHAT IT MEASURES: The TSI Belief Scale is intended to measure disruptions in beliefs about self and others which arise from psychological trauma or from vicarious exposure to trauma material through psychotherapy or other helping relationships. The scale is intended to provide a quick (15 Minute) screening instrument for clinicians questioning the possibility of a trauma history in their clients, as well as indicating specific psychological areas requiring attention in the psychotherapy process. It is also intended, in conjunction with other measures, to diagnose the existence of vicarious traumatization

Sample Items:

1	2	3	4	5	6
Disagree Strongly	Disagree	Disagree Somewhat	Agree Somewhat	Agree	Agree Strongly

_____1. I believe I can protect myself if my thoughts become self-destructive.

_____2. People shouldn't place too much trust in their friends.

_____3. I can't work effectively unless I'm the leader.

REFERENCES:

Mas, K., & Pearlman, L.A. (manuscript in preparation). Disrupted Schemata in *Adult Survivors of Childhood Sexual Abuse.*

McCann, I.L., & Pearlman, L.C. (1990a). Vicarious Traumatization: A framework for understanding the psychological impact of working with victims, *Journal of Traumatic Stress*, 3, 131-150.

McCann, I.E., & Pearlman, L.A. (1990b). *Psychological trauma and the Adult Survivor: Theory, Therapy and Transformation.* New York: Brunner/Mazel.

McCann, I.L., Sakheim, D.K., & Abrahamson, D.J. (1988). Trauma and victimization: A model of psychological adaptation. *The Counseling Psychologist*, 12 (4), 531-594.

Pearlman, L.A., & Mac Ian, P.S. (manuscript in preparation). *The TSI Belief Scale: Data from four criterion groups*.

Pearlman, L.A., & Mac Ian, P., Mas, K., Stamm, B.H., Bieber, S. (October 24, 1992). "Understanding disrupted schemas: The relation among therory, psychotherapy, and research." Presentation at the annual meeting of The International Society for Traumatic Stress Studies, Los Angeles, CA.

Stamm, B.H., Bieber, S.L., & Pearlman, L.A. (October 26, 1991). "A preliminary report on scale construction and generalizability of the TSI Belief Scale." Paper presented at the annual meeting of The International Society for Traumatic Stress Studies, Washington, D.C.

INSTRUMENT CONTACT NAME: Laurie Anne Pearlman, Ph.D.

Address: The Traumatic Stress Institute
                                                          22 Morgan Farms Drive
                                                          South Windsor, CT 06074-1369
Phone: 203-644-2541
Fax: 203-644-6891
Email: CAAPTSI@AOL.com

Women's War-Time Stressor Scale

TYPE OF POPULATION: Women who have served in military or civilization capacities in a war zone or during war time.

COST: None

WHAT IT MEASURES: The scale is a self-report measure of various stressors experienced during war time.

INSTRUMENT CONTENT SUMMARY: While instruments have effectively measured war zone stress in males, the stressors specific to women in a war zone have not been fully addressed. This scale encompasses potential stressors related to the quality of care provided or observed, significant interpersonal difficulties/discriminatory experiences as a woman and/or minority, exposure to severe physical and environmental stressors (including threat to life), and the catastrophic exposure to end of-life events, that is situations specifically involving the dying and dead.

Sample Items:

1. How often did you observe patients die because of lack of equipment or personnel?

> 0=Never
> 1=1-2 times
> 2=3-12 times
> 3=13-50 times
> 4=51 or more times

2. What percentage of the time did you make critical or life-threatening errors in your work because of excessive fatigue or workload (i.e., as compared to the average level of fatigue or workload in the war zone)?

> 0=Never
> 1=Between 1-25%
> 2=Between 26-50%
> 3=Between 51-75%
> 4=>75%

3. What percentage of the women or men you know, or were close to, were killed, wounded, or MIA?

0=Never
1=Between 1-25%
2=Between 26-50%
3=Between 51-75%
4=>75%

INSTRUMENT CONTACT NAME: Jessica Wolfe, Ph.D.

Address:

National Center for PTSD
Women's Health Sciences Division
(116B-2)
VAMC 150 S. Huntington Avenue
Boston, MA 02130

Phone: 617-232-9500 x5916 or x4145
Fax: 617-278-4515

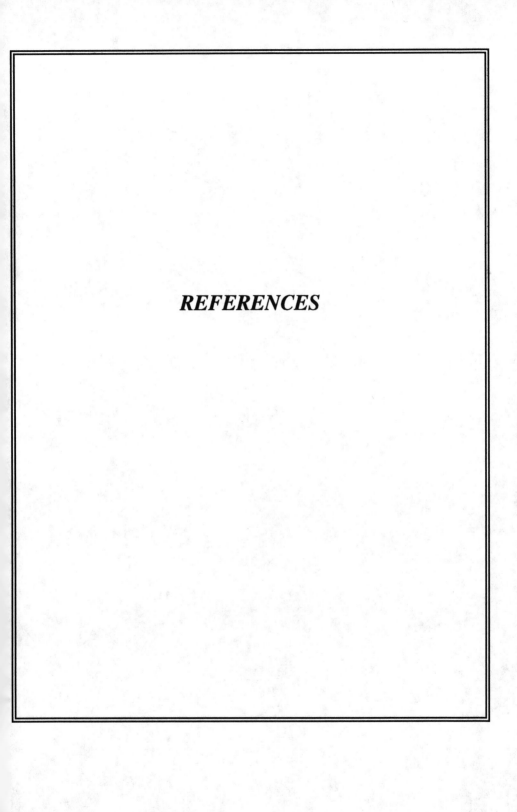

REFERENCES

REFERENCES

Aldwin, C. (1994). Coping with traumatic stress. In C. Aldwin (Ed.), stress, coping and development: an interactive perspective. New York: Guilford Press.

Alfaro, R. (1986). application of nursing process: A step-by-step guide. Philadelphia, PA: J.B. Lippincott.

American Psychiatric Association. (1987). Diagnostic and statistical manual for mental disorders, (Rev. 3rd ed), Washington, DC: American Psychiatric Association.

American Psychiatric Association. (1995). Diagnostic and statistical manual for mental disorders, (4th ed.) Washington, DC: American Psychiatric Association. Author.

American Red Cross. (1992). Disaster manual on health services, I. New York: Author.

Andrews, G., Tennant, C., Hewson, D.M., & Vaillant, G.E. (1978). Life event stress, social support, coping style and risk of psychological impairment. Journal of Nervous Mental Disorders, 66, 307-316.

Antonovsky, A. (1979). Health, stress, and coping. San Francisco: Jossey-Bass.

Antonovsky, A. (1986). Intergenerational networks and transmitting the sense of coherence. In N. Datan, A. Green, & W. Reese, (Eds.). Life-span development psychology: intergenerational relations. Hillside, NJ: Lawrence Erlbaum and Associates.

Antonovsky, A. (1987). Unraveling the mystery of health: how people manage stress and stay well. San Francisco: Jossey-Bass.

Antonovsky, A. (1990a). Pathways leading to successful coping and health. In M. Rosenbaum (Ed.), Learned resourcefulness: on coping skills, self-control, and adaptive behavior. New York: Springer.

Antonovsky, A. (1990b). Personality and health: testing the sense of coherence model. In H. Friedman (Ed.), Personality and disease. New York: John Wiley & Sons.

Antonovsky, A. (1990c). The salutogenic model of health. In R. Ornstein & C. Swencionis (Eds.), The healing brain: a scientific reader. New York: Guilford Press.

Antonovsky, A. (1993). The implications of salutogensis: an outsider's view. In A. Turnbull, J. Patterson, S. Behr, D. Murphy, et. al. (Eds.), Cognitive coping, families and disability. Baltimore: Paul H. Brookes Publishing.

Antonovsky, A. (1991). The structural success sources of salutogenic strengths. In C. Cooper & R. Payne (Eds.), Personality and stress: individual differences in the stress process. England: John Wiley & Sons.

Applebaum, D.R. and Burns, G.L. (1991). Unexpected childhood death: Post-traumatic stress disorder in surviving siblings and parents. Journal of Clinical Child Psychology, 20, 114-120.

Arata, C.M., Saunders, B.E., & Kilpatrick, D.G. (1991). Concurrent validity of a crime-related Post-traumatic stress disorder scale for women within this symptom checklist-90-revised. Violence and Victims, 3, 191-199.

Armstrong, K., O'Callahan, W. & Marmare, C.R. (1991). Debriefing Red Cross disaster personal: The multiple stressor debriefing model. Journal of Traumatic Stress, 4, 581-594.

Arrien, A. (1993). The Four Fold Way. San Francisco: Harper.

Austin, L. (Ed). (1992). Responding to disaster: a guide for mental health professionals. Washington, DC: American Psychiatric Press.

Axelrod, S., Schnipper, O.C., & Rau, H.H. (1980). Hospitalized offspring of Holocaust survivors. Bulletin of the Meninger Clinic, 44 (10), 1-14.

Baker, R. (1992). Psychosocial consequences for tortured refugees seeking asylum and refugee status in Europe. In M. Basoglu (Ed.), Torture and its consequences. Cambridge, England: Cambridge University Press.

Barath, A. (1994). Personal Communication with B. Kazanis.

Barath, A. (1993). Children's self-healing from traumatic war experiences via artistic expression: An art-therapeutic call for children's rights to live and grow in peace. Proposed Exhibition Catalogue. Zagreb, Croatia.

Bartone, P., Ursano, R., Wright, K., & Ingraham, L. (1989). The Impact of military air disaster on the health of assistance workers: A prospective study. Journal of Nervous and Mental Diseases. 177(6), 317-328.

Baum, A.; Fleming, R., & Davidson, L.M. (1983). Emotional, behavioral, and physiological effects of chronic stress at Three Mile Island, Journal of Consulting and Clinical Psychology, 51, 565-572.

Berndt, T.J., & Ladd, G.W. (1989). Peer relationships in child development. New York: Wiley & Sons.

Bettleheim, B. (1984). Afterward to C. Vegh. I didn't say goodbye. R. Schwartz, Translator. New York: E.P. Dutton.

Blake, D.D., Weathers, F., Nagy, L.M., Kaloupek, Klauhnizer, G., D.G., Charney, D. S. & Keane, T.M. (1990). A clinical rating scale for assessing current and lifetime PTSD: The CAPS-1. The Behavior Therapist, 13, 187-188.

Blake, D.D., Weathers, F.W., Nagy, L.M., Kaloupek, D.G., Gusman, F.D., Charney, D.S. & Keane, T.M. (1995). The development of a Clinician-Administered PTSD Scale. Journal of Traumatic Stress, 8(1), 75-90.

Bloch, E.L. (1993). Psychologists in Croatia work to ease trauma among young war victims. Psychology International, 4(3), 1&6.

Bloch, E.L. (1994). Personal communication with B. Kazanis.

Bolin, R. (1985). Disaster characteristics and psychosocial impacts. In, B. Sowder (Ed.), Disasters and mental health: selected contemporary perspectives. (DHHS Publication No. 85-1421, (3-28). Washington, DC: US Govt. Printing Office.

Booker, J. (1992, Winter). Update on Florida disaster response effort. EMDR Network Newsletter.

Boore, J. (1992, Winter). Update on Florida disaster response. EMDR Network Newsletter.

Borysenko, J. (1993). Vision, creativity and purpose. Presentation at the embodying spirit conference. Orlando, FL.

Brand, S. (1990, fall). Learning from the earthquake. Whole Earth Review, 2-15.

Bradburn, N.M. (1969). The Structure of Psychological Well-being. Chicago: Aldine.

Brende, J.O. (1990). Trauma recovery for victims and survivors: Twelve step workbook for readers and participants. Columbus, GA: Trauma Recovery Publications.

Brende, J.O. (1993). A 12-step recovery program for victims of traumatic events. In J.P. Wilson & B. Raphael (Eds.), International Handbook of Traumatic Stress Syndrome. (pp 867-877). New York: Bruner/Mazel.

Brende, J.O. (1994). A twelve theme psychoeducational program for victims and survivors. In M.B. Williams, & J. Sommer (Eds.), Handbook of Post-traumatic Therapy. (pp 421-439). Westport, CT: Greenwood Press.

Brende, J.O. (1991). Acute trauma debriefing: special focus - Law enforcement & police chaplains: Twelve step workbook for leaders and participants. Columbus, GA: Trauma Recovery Publications.

Brende, J.O. (1992). Twelve themes & spiritual steps workbook. Columbus, GA: Trauma Recovery Publications.

Breslau, N., Davis, G.C., Andreski, P., & Peterson, E. (1991). Traumatic events and post traumatic stress disorder in an urban population of young adults. Archives of General Psychiatry, 48, 216-222.

Burgess, A.W., McCausland, M.P. & Wolpert, W.P. (1981). Children's drawings as indicators of sexual trauma. Perspectives in Psychiatric Care, 19, 50-58.

Burk, J., & Judd, L. (1990). Mental health extramureal research support programs. Washington, DC: National Institute of Mental Health.

Capler, A. (1964). Principles of Preventative Psychiatry. New York: Basic Books.

Carr, C. (1993). Death and near-death: A comparison of Tibetan and Euro-American experiences. The Journal of Transpersonal Psychology, 25, 59-110.

Cohen, B. (1993). Sensing, feeling and action: The experiential anatomy of body-mind centering. Amherst, MA: School for Body-Mind Centering.

Cohen, J. (1960). A coefficient of agreement for normal scales. Educational and Psychological Measurement, 20, 37-46.

Cohen R.R. & Ahearn, F.L. (1980). Handbook for mental health care of disaster victims. Baltimore: John Hopkins University Press.

Cohen, R.E. (1992). Training mental health professionals to work with families in diverse cultural contexts. In L.S. Austin (Ed.), Responding to disaster: A guide for mental health professionals. Washington, DC: American Psychiatric Press.

Colodzin, B. (1993). How to survive trauma: A program for war veterans and survivors of rape, assault, abuse or environmental disasters. Barrytown, NY: Station Hill Press.

Danieli, Y. (1980). The aging survivors of the Holocaust: Discussion on the achievement of intergenerational aging survivors of the Nazi Holocaust. Journal of Geriatric Psychiatry, 14 (2), 191-209.

Danieli, Y. (1981a). Families of survivors of the Nazi Holocaust some short and long-term effect. In C.D. Speilberger, I.G. Sarason & N. Milgram (Eds.), Stress and anxiety. (Vol 8). New York: McGraw-Hill/Hemisphere.

Danieli, Y. (1981b). On the achievement of integration of aging survivors of the Nazi Holocaust. Journal of Geriatric Psychiatry, 14(2), 191-210.

Danieli, Y. (1982a). Therapists' difficulties in treating survivors of the Nazi Holocaust and their children. (Doctoral dissertation, New York University, 1981). University Microfilms International, No. 949-904.

Danieli, Y. (1984). Psychotherapists' participation in the conspiracy of silence about the Holocaust. Psychoanalytic Psychology, 1(1), 23-42.

Danieli, Y. (1985). The treatment and prevention of long-term effects and intergenerational transmission of victimization: A lesson learned from Holocaust survivors and their children. In C.R. Figley (Ed.), Trauma and its wake (pp 295-313). New York: Brunner/Mazel.

Danieli, Y. (1988). Confronting the unimaginable: Psychotherapists' reactions to victims of the Nazi Holocaust. In J.P. Wilson, Z. Harel & B. Kahana (Eds.). Human adaptation to extreme stress (pp. 219-238). New York: Plenum.

Danieli, Y. (1989). Mourning in survivors and children of survivors of the Nazi Holocaust: The role of group and community modalities. In D.R. Dietrich & P.C. Shabad (Eds.), The problem of loss and mourning: Psychoanalytic perspectives (pp 427-460). Madison, WI: International Universities Press.

Danieli, Y. (1993). The diagnostic and therapeutic use of multi-generational family tree in working with survivors and children survivors of the Nazi Holocaust. In J.P. Wilson & B. Raphael (Eds.), The international handbook of traumatic stress syndromes. (Stress and coping series) (pp. 889-898). New York: Plenum Publishing.

Danieli, Y. (1994a). Countertransference: trauma and training. In, J.P. Wilson & J. Lindy (Eds.), Countertransference in the treatment of Post-traumatic stress disorder (pp. 368-388). New York: Guilford Press.

Danieli, Y. (1994b). Countertransference and trauma: Self healing and training issues. In M.B. Williams & J.F. Sommer, Jr. Handbook of Post-traumatic therapy. Westport, CT: Greenwood/Praeger Publishing.

Danieli, Y. (1994c). Resilience and hope. In G. Lejeune (Ed.), Children worldwide. Geneva: International Catholic Child Bureau. (in press).

Danieli, Y. (1994d). As survivors age - Part I. National Center for Post Traumatic Stress Disorder Clinical Quarterly, 4(1), 1-7.

Danieli, Y., & Krystal, J.H. (1989). The initial report of the presidential task force on curriculum, education and training for the society for traumatic stress studies. Chicago: The Society for Traumatic Stress Studies.

Davidson, A. (1979). Air disaster coping with stress: A program that worked. Police Stress, 1(2), 20-22.

de La fuente, D., (1994). Temblor shook more than just structures. Modern Healthcare, 24, 1, 52.

Department of Humanitarian Affairs, (DHA). (1993). Strategic aspects of geological and seismic disaster management and disaster scenario planning. Selected presentations made at training seminars in Moscow, Alma-Ata, & Frunze, October 1991, 1990. Geneva: United Nations.

Derogatis, L.R. (1977). SCL-90 administration, scoring & procedure manual for the R (rev.). Baltimore: Johns Hopkins University School of Medicine.

Derogatis, L.R., & Cleary, P.A. (1977a). Factorial invariance across gender for the primary symptom dimensions of the SCL-90. British Journal of Social and Clinical Psychology, 16, 347-356.

Derogatis, L.R. & Cleary, P.A. (1977b). Confirmation of the dimensional structure of the SCL-90: A study in construct validation. Journal of Clinical Psychology, 33, 981-989.

Derogatis, L.R. & Melisaratos, N. (1983). The Brief Symptom Inventory: an introductory report. Psychological Medicine, 13, 595-605.

Derogatis, L.R., (1992). The brief symptom inventory (BSI): Administration, scoring and procedures manual (2nd Ed.). Clinical Psychometric Research, Inc.

Des Pres, T. (1976). The survivor. New York: The Oxford University Press.

Disasters around the world: A global view. (1994). World Conference on Natural Disaster Reduction. Yokohama, Japan, May 23-27. Information paper No. 4.

Disaster Relief Act (1974). U.S. Congress. Public Law 93-288. Seaton, 413.

Dunning, C. & Silva, M. (1981). Disaster-induced trauma in rescue workers. Victimology: An International Journal, 5 (2-4), 287-297.

Dunning, C. (1985). Prevention of stress in disaster workers, In American Psychological Association, Role conflicts and supports for emergency workers. National Institute for Mental Health, Washington, DC: US Government Printing Office.

Dunning, C. (1988). Intervention strategies for emergency workers. In M. Lystad (Ed.), Mental health in mass emergencies: Theory and practice. New York: Brunner/Mazel.

Dyregrov, A. & Mitchell, J.T. (1992). Work with traumatized children - psychological effects and coping strategies. Journal of Traumatic Stress, 5(1), 5-17.

Ebert, M.W. (1986). The mental health disaster team. Beale AFB Disaster Casualty Control Plan, Annex E (10).

Eitenger, L. & Storm, H. (1973). Mortality and morbidity after excessive stress. New York: Humanities Press.

Everstine, D. & Everstine, L. (1993). The trauma response: Treatment for emotional injury. New York: W.W. Norton.

Farborow, N. & Gordon, N. (1981). Manual for child health workers in major disasters. National Institute of Mental Health. Washington, DC: US Government Printing Office.

Fein, E. (1988, December 9). Toll out in tens of thousands from quake in Soviet Armenia. New York Times, 23.

Fernandez, M.R. (1991). How to help children after a disaster: A guidebook for teachers. Alameda County Mental Health Services. FEMA 219.

Figley, C.R. (1985). Trauma and its wake. New York: Brunner/Mazel.

Figley, C.R. (1989). Helping traumatized families. San Francisco: Jossey-Bass.

Fleming, R., Baum, A., Gisriel, M., & Gatchel, R. (1982). Mediating influences of social support on stress at Three Mile Island. Journal of Human Stress, 8, 14-22.

Flexner, S.B. (1993). Random house unabridged dictionary, (2nd ed.). New York: Random House.

Frankl, V.E. (1962). Man's search for meaning. New York: Simon & Schuster.

Frankl, V.E. (1969). The will to meaning. New York: New American Library.

Frankl, V.E. (1978). The unheard cry for meaning. New York: Simon & Schuster.

Frederick, C.J. (1977). Current thinking about crises and psychological interventions in United States disasters. Mass emergencies, 2, 43-50.

Frederick, C.J. (1986). Children traumatized by catastrophic situation. In S. Eth & R. Pynoos (Eds.), Post traumatic stress disorder in children. Washington, DC: American Psychiatric Press.

Freedy, J. R., Saladin, M.F., Kilpatrick, D.G., Resnick, H.S., & Saunders, B.E. (1994). Understanding acute psychological distress following natural disaster. Journal of Traumatic Stress, 7, 2, 257-273.

Forster, P. (1992). Nature and treatment of acute stress reactions. In L. Austin (Ed.). Responding to disaster: A guide for mental health professionals. Washington, DC: American Psychiatric Press.

Funk, S. (1992). Hardiness: A review of theory and research. Health and psychology, 11(5), 335-345.

Gardner, R. (1971). Therapeutic communication with children: The mutual story-telling technique. New York: Science House Publishers.

Gendlin, E. (1978). Focusing. New York: Everest House.

Gergerian, E. (1991, October). Stress inoculation training and biofeedback in PTSD. Paper presented at the Seventh Annual Convention of the National Society for Traumatic Stress Studies, Washington, DC.

Gist, R., & Lubin, B. (Eds.). (1989). Psychological aspects of disaster. New York: John Wiley & Sons.

Gist, R., & Stolz, S.B., (1982). Mental health promotion and the media: Community response to the Kansas City hotel disaster. American Psychologist, 37, 1136-1139.

Glesei, G.C., Green, B.L., & Winget, C. (1981). Prolonged psychological effects of disaster: A study of Buffalo Creek. New York: Academic Press.

Goleman, D.J. (1984). The Buddha on meditation and states of consciousness. In D.H. Shapiro & R.N. Walsh (Eds.), Meditation: classic and contemporary perspectives. New York: Aldine Publishing Company.

Grainger, R.K. (1992, December). Hurricane Andrew disaster response team. EMDR Network Newsletter.

Green, B. L., Grace, M.C., Lindy, J.D., Titchener, J.L., & Lindy, J.G. (1983). Levels of functional impairment following a civilian disaster: The Beverly Hills Supper Club fire. Journal of Consulting Clinical Psychology, 51, 573-580.

Green, B., Lindy, J. & Grace, M. (1990). Buffalo Creek survivors in the second decade: Stability of stress symptoms. American Journal of Orthopsychiatry, 60, 43-54.

Green, P. (1994). Roads down and out for less than a year. Engineering Narrative Report, 232, 5.

Hamilton, M. (1967). Development of a rating scale for primary depressive illness. British Journal of Social and Clinical Psychology, 6, 278-296.

Hamilton, H. (1960). A rating scale for depression. Journal of Neurology, Neurosurgery, and Psychiatry, 23, 56-62.

Hardin, S.B., Weinrich, M., Weinrich, S. Hardin, T.L., & Garrison, C. (1994). Psychological distress of adolescents exposed to Hurricane Hugo. Journal of Traumatic Stress, 7,3, 427-440.

Hartsough, D.M. & Myers, D.G. (1985). Disaster work and mental health: Prevention and control of stress among workers. Center for Mental Health Studies of Emergencies. National Institute of Mental Health. Washington, DC: US Government Printing Office.

Harwood, M. (1991). Art therapy research in England: Impressions of an American art therapist. Art in Psychotherapy, 17(1), 75-79.

Herman, J. (1992). Trauma and recovery. New York: Basic Books.

Hersey, P. & Blanchard, K.H. (1977). Management of organizational behavior: utilizing human resources. (3rd ed.). Englewood Cliffs, NJ: Prentice-Hall.

Hill, W.S. (1994). American Psychiatric Association Affairs Network Coordinator. Personal communication with A. S. Kalayjian.

Horowitz, M. (1986). Stress response syndromes. Northvale, NJ: Jason Aronson.

Horowitz, M., Wilner, W., & Alvarez, W. (1979). Impact of Event Scales: A measure of subjective stress. Psychosomatic Medicine, 41, 209-218.

Hovannisian, R.G. (1969). Armenia on the road to independence. Los Angeles: University of California Press.

Hovannisian, R.G. (Ed.). (1988). The Armenian genocide in perspective. New Brunswick, NJ. Transaction Publishers.

Institute For Armenische Fragen. (1987). The Armenian genocide (Vol. 1). Munich.

Ishkhanian, R. (1989). Badgerazart Badmoutioun Hayotz. (A Pictorial History of Armenians.). Armenian SSR: Arevig Press.

Janoff-Bulman, R. (1992). Shattered assumptions: Towards a new psychology of trauma. New York: Free Press.

Jerazian, L. (1993, Aug.). Psychological techniques of working with earthquake survivors. Presentation at the Glendale Adventist Medical Center, Glendale, CA.

Johnson, O. (Ed.). (1995). 1995 Information please almanac. New York: Houghton Miffin.

Jordan, R.P. (1978). The proud Armenians. National Geographic, 153, 846-873.

Joseph, S.A., Williams, R., Yule, W. & Walker, A. (1992). Factor analysis of the impact of events scale with survivors of two disasters at sea. Personal and Individual Differences, 13, 693-697.

Joseph, S.A., Yule, W., Williams, R. & Hadgkinson. (1993). The herald of free enterprise disaster: Measuring post-traumatic symptoms 30 months on. British Journal of Clinical Psychology, 32, 326-331.

Kalayjian, A.S. (1989). Coping with cancer: The spouse's perspective. Archives of Psychiatric Nursing, III (3), 166-172.

Kalayjian, A.S., et al. (1995). Coping with Ottoman-Turkish genocide. The experience of Armenian survivors. Journal of Traumatic Stress, 9,1, 87-97.

Kalayjian, A.S. (1991a, October). Genocide, earthquake, and ethnic turmoil: Multiple traumas of a nation (abst. 226). Paper presented at the 7th Annual Convention of the International Society for Traumatic Stress Studies: Washington, DC.

Kalayjian, A.S. (1994). Mental health outreach program following the earthquake in
Armenia: Utilizing the nursing process in developing and managing the post-
natural disaster plan. Issues in Mental Health Nursing, 15,6, 533-550.

Kalayjian, A.S. (1994a). Emotional and environmental connections: Impact of the
Armenian earthquake. In E.A. Schuster & C.L. Brown (Eds.), Exploring our
environmental connections. New York: National League for Nursing Press.

Kalayjian, A.S. (1993, June). Politics of developing and managing international mental
health outreach programs in Armenia. Paper presented at the Sigma Theta Tau
International Research Congress, Madrid, Spain.

Kalayjian, A.S. (1991b). Communications with Vasken Manookian in Armenia.

Kalayjian, A.S. (1991c). Meaning in trauma: Impact of the earthquake in Soviet Armenia.
Paper presented at the VIII World Congress of Logotherapy, San Jose, CA.

Kaplan, H.I. & Sadok, B.J. (1991). Synopsis of psychiatry. Baltimore: Williams &
Wilkins.

Kardiner, A. (1959). Traumatic neuroses of war. In S. Arieti (Ed.). American Handbook
of Psychiatry, Vol 1. New York: Basic Books.

Kazanis, B. (1991). Creating ritual: finding and respecting our own ways of grieving.
Creation Spirituality, 7(6), 42-43.

Kazanis, B. (1993). Personal communication with E. Baker.

Kelly, S. (1984, Dec.). The use of art therapy with sexually abused children. Journal of
Psychosocial Nursing and Mental Health Services. 22 (12), 12-18.

Kempen, G.I.J.M. (1992). Psychometric properties of Bradburn's Affect Balance Scale
among elderly persons. Psychological Reports, 70, 638.

Klein. H. & Kogan, I. (1988). Some observations on denial and avoidance in Jewish
Holocaust and post Holocaust experience. In E.L. Edelstein, D.L. Nathanson, &
A.M. Stone (Eds.), Denial: A clarification of concepts and research. New
York: Plenum Press.

Klein-Parker, F. (1988). Dominant attitudes of adult children of Holocaust survivors
toward their parents. In J.P. Wilson, Z. Harel & B. Kahana (Eds.), Human
adaptation to extreme stress. New York: Plenum Press.

Kobasa, S., Maddi, S. & Cahn, S. (1982) Hardiness and health, a prospective study.
Journal of Personality and Social Psychology, 42, 168-177.

Kobasa, S. & Puccetti, M. (1983). Personality and social resources in stress resistance.
Journal of Personality and Social Psychology, 45, 839-850.

Konker, C. (1992). Conceptions of child abuse: A micro and macro perspective.
Dissertation. University of Washington, Seattle, WA. 194-204.

Kubler-Ross, E. (1969). On death and dying. New York: Macmillan Company.

Krystal, H. & Niederland, W.G. (1968). Clinical observations on the survivor syndrome.
In H. Krystal (Ed.), Massive psyche drama. New York: International University
Press.

Kuhn, W., Bell, R.A., Seligson, D., Laufer, S.T. & Linder, J.E. (1988). The tip of the
iceberg: Psychiatric consultation on an orthopedic service. International Journal
of Psychiatry in Medicine, 18, 375-382.

Kupelian, D. (1993). Armenian genocide survivors: Adaptation and adjustment eight decades after massive trauma. (Doctoral dissertation. The American University). University Microfilms International, No. 942271, Vol. 29-02, 0322.

Laube, J., Murphy, S. (1985). Perspectives on disaster recovery. East Norwalk, CT: Appleton-Century-Crofts.

Levick, M., Safran, D., & Levine, A. (1990). Art therapist as expert witnesses: A judge delivers a precedent-setting decision. The Arts in Psychotherapy, 17, 49-53.

Levine, S. (1989). A gradual awakening. New York: Anchor Books.

Liang, J. (1985). A structural integration of the Affect Balance Scale and the life satisfaction index A, Journal of Gerontology. 40, 552-561.

Lifton, R.J., Olsen, E. (1976). The human meaning of total disaster: The Buffalo Creek experience. Psychiatry. 39. 1-17.

Luft, J. (1966). Group process: An introduction to group dynamics. Palo Alto, CA: National Press.

Lyons, J.A. (1991). Strategies for assessing the potential for positive adjustment following trauma. Journal of Traumatic Stress, 4, 93-113.

Lystad, M. (1989). Mental health response to mass emergencies: Theory and Practice. New York: Brunner/Mazel.

Lystad, M. (1986). Disasters and mental health, innovations in service to disaster victims. Washington, DC: American Psychiatric Press.

Maddi, S. & Kobasa, S. (1984). The hardy executive: Health under stress. Homewood, IL: Dow-Jones Irwin.

Mantell, M. (1984). When the badge turns blue. In J. Reese & H. Goldstein (Eds.), Psychological services for law enforcement. Washington, DC: U.S. Government Printing Office.

Maslow, A.H. (1954). Motivation and personality. New York: Harper and Row.

Maslow, A. (1977). The farther reaches of human nature. New York: Esalan Books.

McCann, L. & Pearlman, L.A. (1990). Vicarious traumatization: A framework for understanding the psychological effects of working with victims. Journal of Traumatic Stress, 3, 131-149.

McNiff, S. (1989). Depth psychology of art. Springfield, IL: Charles C. Thomas Publishing.

Meichenbaum, D. (1984). Mental health and world citizenship. Founding document of the World Federation for Mental Health. London, England: WFMH.

Meichenbaum, D. (1985). Stress inoculation training, New York: Pergamon Press.

Meichenbaum, D. (1994). A clinical handbook/practical therapist manual for assessing and treating adults with PTSD. Waterloo, Canada: Institute Press.

Milgram, N., Toubiana, Y., Klingman, A., Raviv, A., & Goldstein, I. (1988). Situational exposure and personal loss in children's acute and chronic stress reactions to a school bus disaster. Journal of Traumatic Stress, 1(3), 339-352.

Mitchell, J., Bray, G. (1990). Emergency services stress: Guidelines for preserving the health and careers of emergency services personnel. Englewood Cliffs, NJ: Prentice-Hall.

Mollica, R., et al. (1973). The effect of trauma and confinement on functional health and mental status of Cambodian living in Thailand-Cambodian border camps. Journal of the American Medical Association, 270(5).

Moos, R. (1986). Coping response inventory. Palo Alto, CA: Veterans Administration Medical Center.

Mosher, L.R., & Burti, L. (1994). Community mental health: A practical guide. New York: W.W. Norton & Company.

Murphy, S.A. (1988). Self-efficacy and social support: Mediators of stress on mental health following a natural disaster. Western Journal of Nursing Research, 9(1), 58-86.

Murray, R., & Zentner, J. (1985). Nursing concepts for health promotion. Englewood Cliffs, NJ: Prentice-Hall.

Nader, K., Pynoos, R., Fairbanks, L., & Frederick, C. (1990). Children's Post-traumatic stress disorder reactions one year after a sniper attack at their school. American Journal of Psychiatry, 147(11), 1526-1530.

National Institute of Mental Health. (1985). Assessment of mental health problems in disaster victims. Special Announcement: MH-86-03. Department of Health and Human Services; Public Health Service: Washington, DC.

National Organization for Victim Assistance. (1991). Community crisis response team training manual. Washington, DC: National Organization for Victim Assistance.

Neale, E. & M. Rosal (1993). What can art therapists learn from the research on projective drawing techniques in children? A review of the literature. Arts in Psychotherapy, (Special Issue), 20 (1), 37-49.

Neiderbach, S. (1994). Personal communication with J. Braak.

Newman, C.J. (1976). Children of disaster: Clinical observations at Buffalo Creek. American Journal of Psychiatry, 133, 306-312.

Nietzsche, F. (1956). Birth of tragedy and other genealogy of morales. Translated by Francis Golffing. New York: Doubleday.

Nordland, R. (1994). Counting the living. Newsweek, CXXIII (4), 36-37.

Ochberg, F.M. (1988). Post traumatic therapy and victims of violence. New York: Brunner/Mazel.

Ochberg, F.M. (1991). Post-traumatic therapy. Psychotherapy, 28, 5-15.

Ogata, S. (1993, February 5). Statement by Mrs. Sadako Ogata, United Nations High Commissioner for Refugees. Roundtable discussion on United Nations. Human Rights Protection of Internally Displaced Persons. Nyon, Switzerland: UN Publications.

Olsen, A. (1993). Body stories. Barrytown, NY: Station Hill Press.

Pan American Health Organization. (1987). Assessing needs in the health sector after floods and hurricanes. Technical paper No. 11. Washington, DC: World Health Organization.

Pan American Health Organization. (1992). Disaster mitigation guidelines for hospitals. Washington, DC: Regional Office of the World Health Organization.

Pan American Health Organization. (1993). Mitigation of disasters in health facilities: General issues (Vol. 1). Washington, DC: Regional Office of the World Health Organization.

Pan American Health Organization. (1993). Mitigation of disasters in health facilities: Administrative issues (Vol. 2). Washington, DC: Regional Office of the World Health Organization.

Pan American Health Organization. (1993). Mitigation of disasters in health facilities: Architectural issues (Vol. 3). Washington, DC: Regional Office of the World Health Organization.

Pan American Health Organization. (1993). Mitigation of disasters in health facilities: Engineering issues (Vol. 4). Washington, DC: Regional Office of the World Health Organization.

Parad, H., Resnik, H., & Parad, L. (1976). Emergency and disaster management: A mental health sourcebook. Bowie, MD: Charles Press Publishers.

Paton, D. (1994). Disaster relief work: An assessment of training effectiveness. Journal of Traumatic Stress, 7,2 257-273.

Phifer, J.F., Kaniasty, K.Z., & Norris, F.H. (1988). The impact of natural disaster on the health of older adults: A multiwave prospective study. Journal of Health and Social Behavior, 29, 65-78.

Pines, D. (1986). Working with women survivors of the Holocaust: Affective experiences in transference and countertransference. International Journal of Psycho-analysis, 67, 295-307.

Prata, C.M., Saunders, B.E., & Kilpatrick, D.G. (1991).

Quarantelli, E.L. (1970). Emergent accommodation groups: Beyond current collective behavior typologies. In T. Sebutai (Ed), Human nature and collective behavior: papers in honor of Herbert Blume (pp. 111-113). Englewood Cliffs, NJ: Prentice-Hall.

Quarantelli, E.L. (1985). An assessment of conflicting views on mental health: The consequences of traumatic events. In C.R. Figley (Ed), Trauma and its wake (pp. 173-215). New York: Brunner-Mazel.

Rappaport, E.A. (1986). Beyond traumatic neurosis: A psychoanalytic study of late reactions to the concentration camp trauma. International Journal of Psychoanalysis, 49, 719-731.

Riordan, R. & A. Verdel. (1991, Nov.). Evidence of sexual abuse in children's art products. School Counselor, 39 (2), 116-121.

Robin. A.A., Harris, J.A. (1962). A controlled comparison of implamtic and electroplexy. Journal of Medical Science, 108, 217-219.

Robins, L.N., Helzer, J.E., Croughan, J., & Ratcliff, K.S. (1981). National Institute of Mental Health diagnostic interview schedule. Archives of General Psychiatry, 38, 318-389.

Robins, L.N., & Smith, E.M. (1983). The diagnostic interview schedule/disaster supplement. St. Louis: Washington University School of Medicine.

Rogers, C.R.. (1957). Client-centered therapy: Its current practice, implications, theory. Boston: Houghton Mifflin.

Rogers, R. (1992, Winter). The future of refugee flows and policies. International Migration Review, 26 (4).

Rogers, N. (1993). The creative connection: Expressive arts as healing. Science and Behavior Books.

Rosenbaum, D., & Post, N.M. (1994). Repairs begin as damage mounts. Engineering Narrative Review, 232, 4, 6-11.

Rosenbaum, D., & McManamy, R. (1994). Isolating the causes of bad buildings behavior. Engineering Narrative Review, 232, 5, 18-22.

Rosenbaum, M. (1990). Learned resourcefulness: On coping skills, self-control, and adaptive behavior. New York: Springer Publishing.

Rozynko, V. & Dondershine, H.E. (1991). Trauma focus group therapy for Vietnam veterans with PTSD. Psychotherapy, 28, 157-161.

Rutter, M., Izard, C.E., & Read, P.B. (1986). Depression in young people: Developmental and clinical perspectives. New York: Guilford Publishing.

Sarafian, A. (1994). United States official documents on the Armenian genocide.(Vol. I): The lower Euphrates. Watertown, MA: Archival Collections on the Armenian Genocide.

Saunders, B.E., Arata, C.M., & Kilpatrick, D.G. (1990). Development of a crime-related post-traumatic stress disorder scale for women within the Symptom Checklist-90-Revised. Journal of Traumatic Stress, 3, 439-448

Schaffer, M.D. (1982). Multidimensional measures of therapist behavior as predictors of outcome. Psychological Bulletin, 92, 670-681.

Schwarzwald, J., Soloman, Z., Weisenberg, M., & Mikulincer, M. (1987). Validation of the Impact of Event Scale for psychological/sequelae of combat. Journal of Consulting and Clinical Psychology, 55, 251-256.

Shapiro, F. (1989a). Efficacy of the eye movement desensitization procedure in the treatment of traumatic memories. Journal of Traumatic Stress Studies, 2, 199-223.

Shapiro, F. (1989b). Eye movement desensitization: A new treatment for Post-traumatic stress disorder. Journal of Behavior Therapy and Experimental Psychiatry, 20, 211-217.

Shapiro, F. (1992). Manual: Eye movement desensitization and reprocessing. (Level I & II). San Jose: EMDR.

Shapiro, F. (1993). Manual: Eye movement desensitization and reprocessing. (Level I & II). San Jose: EMDR.

Shapiro, F. (1995). Eye movement desensitization and reprocessing: Principles, protocols and procedures. New York: Guilford.

Shultz, I.N. (1983). Ubungheft fur das autogene training. New York: Georg. Thieme Verlag, Stuttgart.

Sime, J.D. (1980). The concept of panic. In D. Canter (Ed.), Free and human behavior (pp. 63-81). London: Wiley & Sons.

Simon, P. (1989). U.S. Government should do more to help Armenia rebuild. Journal of Armenian Assembly of America, 16, 3-4.

Slaby, A.E. (1988). After-shock. New York: Random House.

Slaby, A.E., Lieb, J., & Tancredi, L.R. (1981). Handbook of psychiatric disorders. Garden City, NY: Medical Examination Publishing.

Sorensen, J.M. et al. (1987). The impact of hazardous technology: The psycho-social effects of restarting TMI-I. New York: SUNY Press.

Solomon, A., Bleich, A., Shoham, S., Nardi, C., & Kotler, M. (1992). The "Koach" project for treatment of combat-related PTSD: Rationale, aims and methodology. Journal of Traumatic Stress, 5, 175-193.

Sowder, B. (1986). Disasters and mental health, contemporary perspectives. Washington, DC: American Psychiatric Press.

Spitzer, R.L., Williams, J.B.W., Gibbon, M., & First, M.B. (1989). Instruction manual for the Structured Clinical Interview for DSM-III-R, (SCID, 5/1/89 Revision). New York: New York State Psychiatric Institute, Biometrics Research Department.

Spofford, P. J., et al. (1990). School intervention following a critical incident. FEMA, 220.

Spofford, P. J., et al. (1991). Children and trauma: The schools response. Video. California State Department of Mental Health. FEMA.

SPSS-X user's Guide (3rd Ed.) (1988). New York: McGraw-Hill.

Stallins, R. (1973). The community context of crisis management. American Behavioral Scientist, 16, 313-325.

Stember, C.J. (1980). Art therapy: A new use in the diagnosis and treatment of sexually abused children. In Sexual abuse of children: Selected readings (pp 59-63). Washington, D.C: Government Printing House.

Stern, G.M. (1976). The Buffalo Creek disaster. New York: Random House.

Strupp, H.H., Hadley, S.W., & Gomes-Schwartz, B. (1977). Psychotherapy for better or worse: The problem of negative effects. New York: Jason Aronson.

Suinn, R.M., Deffenbacher J.L. (1988). Anxiety management training. The Counseling Psychologist, 16, 31-49.

Sullivan, W. (1988, December). Pressing rock masses mark center of quake. The New York Times, 6.

Sullivan, G. (1993). Towards clarification of convergent concepts: Sense of coherence, will to meaning, locus of control, learned helplessness and hardiness. Journal of Advanced Nursing, 18(11), 1772-1778.

Symonds, M. (1980). The "second injury" to victims. Evaluation and change. (Special Issue), 36-38.

Takooshian, H., Kalayjian, A.S., & Melkonian, E. (1993). The Soviet Union and post-Soviet era. In L.L. Adler (Ed.), International handbook on gender roles (pp. 324-357). Westport, CT: Greenwood Press.

Talbot, A., Manton, M. & Dunn, P.J. (1992). Debriefing the debriefers: An intervention strategy to assist psychologists after a crisis. Journal of Traumatic Stress, 4, 45-62.

Talbot, A., Manton, M. & Dunn, P.J. (1992). Debriefing the debriefers: An intervention strategy to assist psychologists after a crisis. Journal of Traumatic Stress, 5, (1), 45-62.

Taylor, A. & Fraser, A. (1984). Architecture, disaster and human stress. Ekistics: The problem and science of human settlement, 308, 445-451.

Terr, L.C. (1989). Family anxiety after traumatic events. Journal of Clinical Psychiatry, 50, 11, 15-19.

Thompson, W. (1981). The time falling bodies take to light: Mythology, sexuality, and the origins of culture. New York: St. Martin's Press.

Tierney, K.J. (1986, October). Disaster and mental health: A critical look at knowledge and practice. Paper presented at the Italy-United States Conference on Disaster Research, University of Delaware, Disaster Research Center, Newark, Delaware.

Tierney, K.J. (1986). The social and community contexts of disaster. In R. Gist and B. Lubin (Eds.), Psychosocial aspects of disaster (pp. 11-39). New York: John Wiley & Sons.

Tierney, K.J., & Baisden, B. (1979). Crisis intervention programs for disaster victims: A source-book and manual for smaller communities. (Publication No. ADM 79-675). Washington, DC: Department of Health, Education and Welfare.

Titchener J.L., & Kapp F.T. (1976). Family and character change at Buffalo Creek. American Journal of Psychiatry, 133, 295-299.

Ulman, E. & Levy, B. (1992). Art therapists as diagnosticians. American Journal of Art Therapy, 30 (2), 117-118.

Ulman, E. & Dachinger, P. (1975). Art therapy in theory and practice. New York: Schocken Books.

Ulman, A.C. (1981). Health impact of the Three Miles Island accident. In T.H. Moss & D.L. Sills (Eds.), The Three Miles Island nuclear accident: Lessons and implications. (p. 375) (Vol 365). Annals of the New York Academy of Sciences.

United Nations Environment Program. (1993-1994). Environment data report. Oxford, England: Blackwell Publishers.

Ursano, R.J., McCaughey, B.G., & Fullerton, C.S. (1994). Individual and community response to trauma and disaster. New York: Cambridge University Press.

U.S. Agency for International Development and U.S. Department of State (1991). Discussion paper: Health care problems of the Soviet Union.

U.S. Department of Health and Human Service. (1986). Training manual for human service workers in major disasters. Rockville, MD: National Institute of Mental Health.

U.S. National Committee for the Decade for Natural Disaster Reduction: commission on Geosciences, Environment and Resources: National Research Council. (1994). Facing the challenge: The U.S. national report to the IDNDR World Conference on National Disaster Reduction. Yokohama, Japan, May 23-27, 1994. Washington, DC: National Academy Press.

van der Kolk, B. (1987). The role of the group in the origin and resolution of the trauma response. In B. van der Kolk (Ed.). Psychological trauma. Washington, DC: American Psychiatric Association Press.

van der Kolk, B.A. (1984). The psychobiology of the trauma response: Hyperarousal, constriction and addition. In B.A. van der Kolk (Ed) Psychological trauma. Washington, DC: American Psychiatric Press.

Wadson, H. (1975). Is interpretation of sexual symbolism necessary? Art Psychotherapy, 2 (3-4), 233-239.

Walker, B. (1991, Apr. 5). Armenia at crossroads. (television news broadcast). Los Angeles: CBS News.

288

Walker, L. (1994). Listening to the children. Presentation at the juvenile welfare board. St. Petersburg, Fl.

Wagner, M. (1981). Trauma counseling for police officers. In R. Thomlinson (Ed), Perspectives in industrial social work practice. Otawa, Canada, Family Service Canada. See also Wagner, M. (1979). Stress debriefing, flight 191. Chicago Police Star, August, 4-7 and Wagner, M. (1980). Airline disaster: A stress debrief program for police. Police Stress, 2(1), 16-20.

Warheit, G.J. (1976). Similarities and differences. Mass Emergencies, 1, 131-137.

Weiss, D. (1993). Structured clinical interview techniques. In Wilson, J.P., & Raphael, B. (Eds.). International handbook of traumatic stress syndromes. New York: Plenum Press.

Williams, P., Wiebe, D., & Smith, T. Coping processes as mediators of the relationship between hardiness and health. Journal of Behavioral Medicine, 15(3), 237-255.

Wilson, J. P. & J. Lindy (Eds.). (1994). Countertransference in the treatment of post-traumatic stress disorder. New York: Guilford Press.

Williams, T. (1987). Post-traumatic stress disorder: A handbook for clinicians. Cincinnati, OH: Disabled American Veterans.

Williams, T. (1994). Personal communication with J. Braak.

Wilson, J.P., Harel, Z., & Kahana, B. (Eds.). (1989). Human adaptation to extreme stress. New York: Plenum Publishers.

Wilson, H.S., & Kneisl, C.B. (1983). Psychiatric Nursing (2nd Ed.). Redding, MA: Addison Wesley Publishers.

Winnicott, D.W. (1965). The maturational process and the facilitating environment. London, England: Hogarth Press.

Wojcik, J. (1994). Insurers tallying losses. Business Insurance, 28, 7, 2-4.

Wolpe, J. (1982). The practice of behavior therapy. New York: Pergamon Press.

Wright, J.W. (Ed), (1995). The universal almanac 1995. Kansas City, MO: Andrews & McMeel.

Yalom I.D. (1975). The theory and practice of group psychotherapy (2nd Ed.). New York: Basic Books.

Yung, C.G. (1959). The archetypes of the collective unconscious. In The collected works of C.G. Yung. New York: Princeton University Press.

Zabora, J.R., Smith-Wilson, R., Fetting, J.H. & Engerline, J.P. (1990). An efficient method for psychosocial screening of cancer patients. Psychosomatics, 31, 192-196.

Zelman, D., & Metrick, S. (1993). Art from ashes. Oakland, CA: Oakland Arts Council.

Zilberg, N.J., Weiss, D.S., & Horowitz, M.J. (1982). Impact of Event Scale: A cross-validation study and some empirical evidence supporting a conceptual model of stress response syndromes. Journal of Consulting and Clinical Psychology, 50, 407-414.

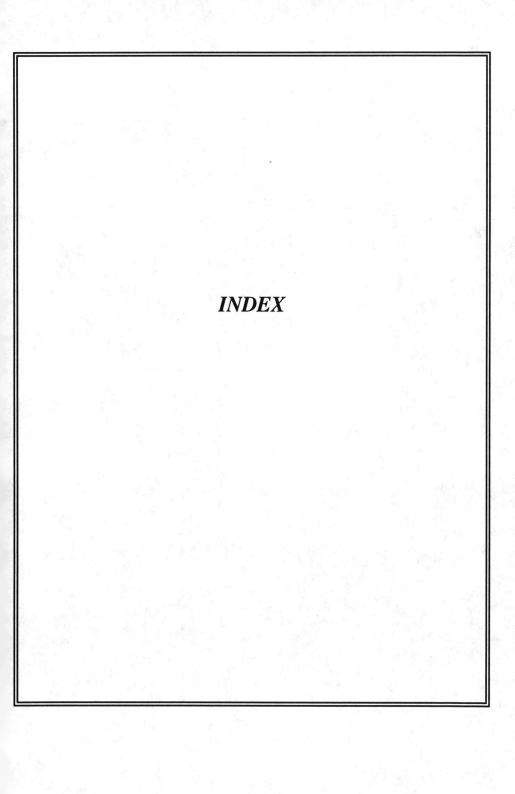

INDEX

trauma volunteers
    debriefing, 91
    preparing, 150
    preparing - celebration, 156
    preparing - exclusion Criteria, 153
    preparing - follow-up, 156
    preparing - inclusion criteria, 152
    preparing - interview, 151
    preparing - orientation, 87
    selecting, 150
tropical storms, 1
tsunamis, 17
typhoons in Japan, 1

—U—

United Nations, 1
    International Decade for Natural Disaster
        Reduction (IDNDR), 1
    Members of, 8
    National Committee Report, 9
    UNICEF, 112
    World Conference on Natural Disaster
        reduction - Japan, 8
United States, 8, 145
United States Geological Survey - National
    Earthquake Information Center, 8
United States National Weather Service, 19

—V—

Valley Fever, 47
victims, 24, 41, 63
    self-help groups, 113, 131, 162
    themes of recovery, 162
volcanoes, 21, 220
volunteers
    see also trauma volunteers, 150
voluntees
    definition, 21
vulnerability, 27

—W—

warning systems, 9
    in Armenia, 9
    United States, 9
wellness, 26, 150, 177, 178, 179, 181, 183
World Federation for Mental Health
    (WFMH), 227
World Health Organization (WHO), 1, 13,
    149, 153
    see also Pan American Health
        Organization (PAHO), 13, 28, 149,
        221

—Y—

Yerevan, 38, 57

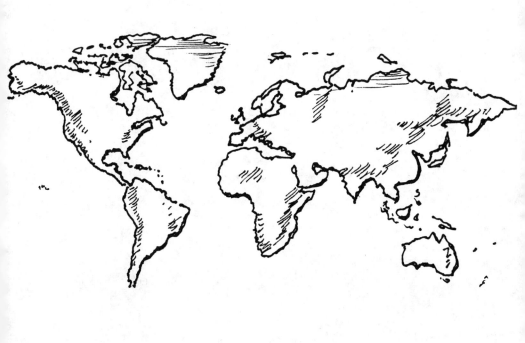